Management of Gastric Cancer

Guest Editor

NEAL WILKINSON, MD

SURGICAL ONCOLOGY
CLINICS OF NORTH AMERICA

www.surgonc.theclinics.com

Consulting Editor
NICHOLAS J. PETRELLI, MD

January 2012 • Volume 21 • Number 1

SAUNDERS an imprint of ELSEVIER, Inc.

W.B. SAUNDERS COMPANY
A Division of Elsevier Inc.

1600 John F. Kennedy Boulevard • Suite 1800 • Philadelphia, PA 19103-2899

http://www.theclinics.com

SURGICAL ONCOLOGY CLINICS OF NORTH AMERICA Volume 21, Number 1
January 2012 ISSN 1055-3207, ISBN-13: 978-1-4557-3940-0

Editor: Jessica McCool

Surgical Oncology Clinics of North America (ISSN 1055-3207) is published quarterly by Elsevier Inc., 360 Park Avenue South, New York, NY 10010-1710. Months of publication are January, April, July, and October. Business and Editorial Offices: 1600 John F. Kennedy Blvd., Ste. 1800, Philadelphia, PA 19103-2899. Customer Service Office: 3251 Riverport Lane, Maryland Heights, MO 63043. Periodicals postage paid at New York, NY and additional mailing offices. Subscription prices are $263.00 per year (US individuals), $386.00 (US institutions) $130.00 (US student/resident), $302.00 (Canadian individuals), $480.00 (Canadian institutions), $186.00 (Canadian student/resident), $377.00 (foreign individuals), $480.00 (foreign institutions), and $186.00 (foreign student/resident). Foreign air speed delivery is included in all *Clinics* subscription prices. All prices are subject to change without notice. **POSTMASTER**: Send address changes to *Surgical Oncology Clinics of North America*, Elsevier Health Science Division, Subscription Customer Service, 3251 Riverport Lane, Maryland Heights, MO 63043. **Customer Service: 1-800-654-2452 (US and Canada). 314-447-8871 (outside U.S. and Canada). Fax: 314-447-8029. E-mail: journalscustomerservice-usa@elsevier.com** (for print support); **journalsonline support-usa@elsevier.com** (for online support).

Reprints. For copies of 100 or more, of articles in this publication, please contact the Commercial Reprints Department, Elsevier Inc., 360 Park Avenue South, New York, New York 10010-1710. Tel. 212-633-3813; Fax: 212-462-1935; E-mail: reprints@elsevier.com.

Surgical Oncology Clinics of North America is covered in *MEDLINE/PubMed (Index Medicus)* and *EMBASE/ Excerpta Medica, Current Contents/Clinical Medicine, and ISI/BIOMED.*

Printed and bound by CPI Group (UK) Ltd, Croydon, CR0 4YY
Transferred to Digital Print 2012

Contributors

CONSULTING EDITOR

NICHOLAS J. PETRELLI, MD
Bank of America Endowed Medical Director, Helen F. Graham Cancer Center at Christiana Care Health System, Newark, Delaware; Professor of Surgery, Thomas Jefferson University, Philadelphia, Pennsylvania

GUEST EDITOR

NEAL WILKINSON, MD
Associate Professor of Surgery, University of Buffalo, State University of New York; Attending Surgeon, Department of Surgical Oncology, Roswell Park Cancer Institute, Buffalo, New York

AUTHORS

JOSEPH J. BENNETT, MD, FACS
Helen F. Graham Cancer Center, Department of Surgery, Christiana Care Health Services, Newark, Delaware

VANESSA R. BLAIR, FRACS, PhD
Lecturer in Surgery, Department of Surgery, Faculty of Medicine and Health Sciences, University of Auckland, Auckland, New Zealand; Department of Surgery, Whangarei Base Hospital, Whangarei, New Zealand

IAN CHAU, MD
Royal Marsden Hospital, London; Department of Medicine, Royal Marsden Hospital, Sutton, Surrey, United Kingdom

DAVID CUNNINGHAM, MD
Professor, Royal Marsden Hospital, London; Department of Medicine, Royal Marsden Hospital, Sutton, Surrey, United Kingdom

RAMI EL ABIAD, MD
Assistant Professor of Medicine, Division of Gastroenterology and Hepatology, University of Iowa Hospitals and Clinics, Iowa City, Iowa

HENNING GERKE, MD
Associate Professor of Medicine, Division of Gastroenterology and Hepatology; Medical Director, Diagnostic and Therapeutic Unit, Digestive Disease Center, University of Iowa Hospitals and Clinics, Iowa City, Iowa

DAVID H. HARPOLE Jr, MD
Professor, Division of Cardiovascular and Thoracic Surgery, Department of Surgery, Duke University Medical Center, Durham, North Carolina

HISAKAZU HOSHI, MD
Clinical Associate Professor, Surgical Oncology and Endocrine Surgery, Department of Surgery, University of Iowa Hospitals and Clinics, Iowa City, Iowa

TOSHIHISA HOSOYA, MD
Digestive Disease Center, Showa University Northern Yokohama Hospital, Yokohama, Japan

SCOTT A. HUNDAHL, MD, FACS, FSSO, FAHNS
Professor of Clinical Surgery, UC Davis; Chief of Surgery, VA Northern California Health Care System, Sacramento VA at Mather, Mather, California

HARUO IKEDA, MD
Digestive Disease Center, Showa University Northern Yokohama Hospital, Yokohama, Japan

HARUHIRO INOUE, MD, PhD, FASGE
Professor of Medicine, Showa University International Training Center for Endoscopy (SUITE), Digestive Disease Center, Showa University Northern Yokohama Hospital, Yokohama, Japan

VIKRAM K. JAIN, FRACP
Royal Marsden Hospital, London, United Kingdom; Department of Medicine, Royal Marsden Hospital, Sutton, Surrey, United Kingdom

NIKHIL I. KHUSHALANI, MD
Assistant Professor of Oncology, Department of Medicine, Roswell Park Cancer Institute, Buffalo, New York

SHIN-EI KUDO, MD, PhD
Professor of Medicine, Director, Digestive Disease Center, Showa University Northern Yokohama Hospital, Yokohama, Japan

MANABU ONIMARU, MD, PhD
Digestive Disease Center, Showa University Northern Yokohama Hospital, Yokohama, Japan

MATTHEW S. RUBINO, MD
Helen F. Graham Cancer Center, Department of Surgery, Christiana Care Health Services, Newark, Delaware

MITSURU SASAKO, MD
Professor, Chairman, Department of Surgery, Hyogo College of Medicine, Nishinomiya, Hyogo, Japan

VIVIAN E. STRONG, MD, FACS
Associate Professor of Surgery, Associate Attending Surgeon, Gastric and Mixed Tumor Service, Department of Surgery, Memorial Sloan-Kettering Cancer Center, Weill Medical College of Cornell University, New York, New York

MICHITAKA SUZUKI, MD
Digestive Disease Center, Showa University Northern Yokohama Hospital, Yokohama, Japan

BETTY C. TONG, MD, MHS
Assistant Professor, Division of Cardiovascular and Thoracic Surgery, Department
of Surgery, Duke University Medical Center, Durham, North Carolina

AKIRA YOSHIDA, MD, PhD
Digestive Disease Center, Showa University Northern Yokohama Hospital, Yokohama,
Japan

Contents

> Gastric cancer is common and is a cause of severe morbidity and mortality. Early diagnosis can improve the chances of cure and prolong survival because prognosis is inversely related to the disease stage. Endoscopy plays an important role in diagnosis. Emerging adjunct technologies such as image-enhanced endoscopy and magnification endoscopy aid in early cancer detection. Endoscopic ultrasonography is an additional useful tool for preoperative staging. Endoscopy for screening, except for high-risk patients, and outside areas of high prevalence, remains controversial.

> Gastrointestinal stromal tumors (GISTs) are relatively rare mesenchymal tumors located within the submucosa of the GI tract. The defining characteristic of GISTs is the presence of the cell-surface antigen CD117 receptor tyrosine kinase, identified by immunohistochemistry. Currently the only cure for GIST is complete surgical resection. Imatinib has revolutionized the treatment of GISTs and has been used as adjuvant treatment after resection, and as treatment for locally advanced, recurrent, and metastatic GIST. Imatinib resistance has become a significant concern in the treatment of GISTs and other tyrosine kinase inhibitors that target different pathways are currently being studied.

> This article focuses on the diagnosis and management of familial gastric cancer, particularly hereditary diffuse gastric cancer (HDGC). First, existing consensus guidelines are discussed and then the pathology and genetics of HDGC are reviewed. Second, patient management is covered, including surveillance gastroscopy, prophylactic total gastrectomy, and management of the risk of breast cancer.

> The quality of surgical treatment is a major determinant of cancer treatment outcomes; however, controlling surgical quality is a difficult task.

Surgical treatment of gastric cancers, and especially the benefits of nodal dissection, has been a topic of debate and no consensus has been reached to date. The D2 nodal dissection defined, standardized, and practiced in Japan is a technically challenging procedure but carries better locoregional disease control. This article reviews the current definition of D1, D1 plus, and D2 nodal dissections, as well as the nodal dissection technique, indications for its modification, and the learning curve.

Several guidelines are used for cancer therapy throughout the world. The Japan Gastric Cancer Association guideline, whereby standard surgery for T2 to T4 curable gastric cancer is defined as more than two-thirds gastrectomy with D2 dissection, are widely followed, with further data being gathered from either single institutions or nationwide registry. In the East, D2 dissection shows much better results than less extended surgery followed by adjuvant treatment. Adjuvant chemotherapy without radiotherapy shows significantly better survival results than surgery alone only when D2 dissection is applied. Without good local control, including regional lymph node metastasis, the cure rate cannot be high.

To optimize the therapeutic value of an operation for cancer, surgeons must weigh survival value against mortality/morbidity risk. As a result of several prospective, randomized trials, many surgeons feel that international opinion has reached a consensus. Reflexively radical surgical hubris has certainly given way to a more nuanced, customized approach to this disease. But issues remain. This article critically reviews existing data and emphasizes areas of continued controversy.

Radical surgery offers the only chance of cure for patients with operable gastric cancer; however, outcomes remain generally poor due to a high rate of relapse post gastric surgery. Multimodality therapy using chemotherapy, radiation or a combination of both have been evaluated in different parts of the world to improve outcomes from surgery alone. Perioperative chemotherapy is generally preferred in Europe in contrast to postoperative chemoradiation in the US or adjuvant fluoropyrimidine chemotherapy in East Asia. Regardless of these variations, systemic chemotherapy consistently results in a survival benefit when used in multimodality treatment of operable gastric cancer.

Gastric cancer remains a global public health problem with considerable heterogeneity in pathogenesis and clinical presentation across geographic regions. Improved understanding of the molecular biology of this disease has opened avenues for targeted intervention. An individualized treatment approach is required for optimal management of this cancer. Overcoming resistance to therapy requires combining targeted agents with the traditional options of chemotherapy/radiation therapy, and also targeting more than 1 pathway of carcinogenesis at a time. Encouraging molecular hypothesis and biomarker-driven trials will lead to improved patient outcomes and may eventually enable the therapeutic nihilism associated with gastric cancer to be overcome.

Mucosal cancer in the gastrointestinal tract generally has low risk of lymph node metastasis. Endoscopic mucosal resection (EMR) and endoscopic submucosal dissection (ESD) are techniques of local excision of neoplasia confined to the mucosal layer. Specimens from EMR/ESD contribute to several diagnoses, and histologic results affect treatment decisions. A combined laparoscopic and endoscopic approach to neoplasia with a nonexposure technique allows full-thickness resection of the stomach wall without exposing the gastric lumen to the peritoneal cavity, preventing cancer cell dissemination to the peritoneal cavity. This article reviews EMR/ESD and describes a new full-thickness resection method using the nonexposure technique (CLEAN-NET).

There has been much speculation regarding differences in outcome for patients who have gastric cancer in the Eastern versus Western world. Among other factors, these differences have contributed to a unique cohort of patients and experience in the Western staging/evaluation of gastric cancer and in the application of minimally invasive approaches for treatment. This review summarizes the current state of laparoscopic approaches for the staging and treatment of gastric adenocarcinoma for patients presenting in Western countries, with their associated unique presentation, comorbidities, and outcomes.

Lung cancer is the most common malignancy in the United States and worldwide. In 2011, it is estimated that more than 221,000 people in the United States will be diagnosed with cancer of the lung and bronchus. For patients with early-stage disease, 5-year survival approaches only 50%. Recent advances using molecular, genetic, and proteomic profiling of lung tumors have enabled refining the prognosis for patients with non–small cell lung cancer. With targeted therapies, there is an opportunity to enhance long-term survival. This article discusses several key molecular markers used in the prognostication and treatment of non–small cell lung cancer.

FORTHCOMING ISSUES

April 2012
Sarcomas
John M. Kane III, MD,
Guest Editor

July 2012
Outcomes Research in Surgical Oncology
Clifford Ko, MD,
Guest Editor

October 2012
Laparoscopic Approaches in Oncology
James Fleshman, MD,
Guest Editor

RECENT ISSUES

October 2011
Lung Cancer
Mark J. Krasna, MD,
Guest Editor

July 2011
Surgical Oncology in the Community
Cancer Center
Frederick L. Greene, MD,
Guest Editor

April 2011
Ablative Procedures in Surgical Oncology
Steven A. Curley, MD,
Guest Editor

RELATED INTEREST

Primary Care: Clinics in Office Practice, September 2011 (Vol. 38, Issue 3)
Gastroenterology
James Winger, MD, and Aaron Michelfelder, MD, *Guest Editors*
Available at: http://www.primarycare.theclinics.com/

VISIT THE CLINICS ONLINE!

Access your subscription at:
www.theclinics.com

Foreword

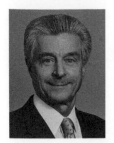

Nicholas J. Petrelli, MD
Consulting Editor

This edition of the *Surgical Oncology Clinics of North America* deals with gastric cancer, although there is a bonus article from the lung cancer issue by Drs Tong and Harpole dealing with molecular markers for incidence, prognosis, and response to therapy. Having said that, the guest editor for this edition of the *Surgical Oncology Clinics of North America* is Neal Wilkinson, MD from the Department of Surgical Oncology at Roswell Park Cancer Institute in Buffalo, New York. Dr Wilkinson has put together 10 articles dealing with many aspects of the diagnosis and treatment of gastric cancer. Included in this edition is an inclusive article by Drs Bennett and Rubino dealing with gastrointestinal stromal tumors of the stomach. A very provocative article by Inoue and colleagues entitled, "Endoscopic Mucosal Resection, Endoscopic Submucosal Dissection, and Beyond: Full-Layer Resection for Gastric Cancer with Non-Exposure Technique (CLEAN-NET)," is also included.

As Dr Wilkinson explains in his preface of the *Surgical Oncology Clinics of North America*, the literature even to this day contains numerous conflicting trials and clinical recommendations for gastric cancer. This is especially true of the tumors that comprise the spectrum of gastric cancer at both a national and an international level and, as stated by Dr Wilkinson, how these differences impact our understanding of the already published literature. Dr Wilkinson has put together a talented group of national and international leaders in the field of gastric cancer, and this edition of the *Surgical Oncology Clinics of North America* will update all physicians in this arena of cancer care.

I would like to take this opportunity to thank Dr Wilkinson and his colleagues for this edition of the *Surgical Oncology Clinics of North America*, and, as I have stated numerous times, this edition, like many others, can be a tremendous educational tool for all young clinicians and investigators in training.

Nicholas J. Petrelli, MD
Helen F. Graham Cancer Center
4701 Ogletown-Stanton Road, Suite 1213
Newark, DE 19713, USA

E-mail address:
npetrelli@christianacare.org

Surg Oncol Clin N Am 21 (2012) xiii
doi:10.1016/j.soc.2011.09.009
1055-3207/12/$ – see front matter © 2012 Elsevier Inc. All rights reserved.

surgonc.theclinics.com

Preface

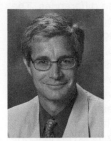

Neal Wilkinson, MD
Guest Editor

Gastric cancer is a fascinating topic for in-depth review and detailed study. Gastric cancer remains far from eradicated despite declining global and national trends. The literature today still poses numerous conflicting trials and clinical recommendations. What are the screening indications and staging studies required to diagnose and treat gastric cancer? What neoplasms comprise the spectrum of gastric cancer at the national and international level and how do these differences impact our understanding of the published literature? What is the optimal surgical approach to this disease: role of minimally invasive staging and resection; the benefit of standard or extended lymphadenectomy? What is the role of adjuvant therapy and what is the optimal sequencing of care? The authors have each been selected and tasked with tackling difficult questions that the practicing surgeon encounters.

We have selected a broad array of national and international leaders to delve into some of the more controversial topics with the goal of understanding when and how to apply the data in the clinical arena. Drs El Abiad and Gerke discuss the role of diagnostic endoscopy in this disease. They explore the future promise of enhanced imaging and ultrasound techniques for early detection and staging. Drs Bennett and Rubino cover the entire spectrum of GIST disease with a clear focus on the extent of surgery and the role of adjuvant treatment. Dr Blair provides an overview of hereditary diffuse gastric cancer, focusing on the genetics, presentation, and treatment she and her colleagues have established through their vast experience in New Zealand. These articles provide a clear and comprehensive overview of the challenges we face when approaching the patient with gastric pathology and lay out clear clinical guidelines for the practicing surgeon.

Controversial topics abound and in this issue; several authors have tackled them head-on with the goal of providing clarity to a literature rich in conflicting results. Dr Hoshi provides a technical overview of the standard D2 resection and demystifies many of the concepts most troubling to surgeons finalizing their training in the United States. No issue on gastric cancer would be complete without dynamic and point and

Surg Oncol Clin N Am 21 (2012) xv–xvi
doi:10.1016/j.soc.2011.09.011
1055-3207/12/$ – see front matter © 2012 Elsevier Inc. All rights reserved.

counterpoint addressing the differences seen between clinical trials and reports published from the east and west. Drs Sasako and Hundahl provide insightful commentary on many of these publications with a focus on understanding these differences. The role of adjuvant therapy in gastric cancer suffers from dramatic regional differences and confusing results. The selected authors, Drs Chau, Jain, Cunningham, and Khushalani, provide a clear understanding of regional practice patterns, important differences between clinical trial comparisons, and future areas of investigation. Next, Dr Inoue and colleagues provide us with a futuristic blend between the capacity and limitations of endoscopy for endoscopic resection with some very novel techniques that blend the best of endoscopy with laparoscopy. Dr Strong examines the role of laparoscopic surgery in both staging and resection of gastric cancer. These articles highlight the need for the surgical oncologist to embrace the role of advanced endoscopy and laparoscopy, yet not lose sight of the importance of surgeon experience and learning curves. The authors tackling these controversial topics have each strived to provide enough material and detail to promote understanding of guidelines and recommendations arising from the literature. It is our hope that these combined articles will enhance the readers' understanding of the published literature and demystify the conflicting published results.

Neal Wilkinson, MD
Department of Surgical Oncology
Roswell Park Cancer Institute
Elm & Carlton Streets
Buffalo, NY 14263, USA

E-mail address:
neal.wilkinson@roswellpark.org

Gastric Cancer: Endoscopic Diagnosis and Staging

Rami El Abiad, MD[a],*, Henning Gerke, MD[a,b]

KEYWORDS

- Gastric cancer • Classification • Screening
- Chromoendoscopy • Endoscopy • Endoscopic ultrasound

Gastric cancer is the fourth most common cancer worldwide, leading to more than 700,000 deaths annually, which is second only to lung cancer.[1,2] Gastric cancer carries a poor prognosis, with 15% to 20% 5-year overall survival even if the disease is limited to the gastric wall.[3] Outcomes are favorable if cancers and their precursors are detected early,[4] and there is a wide window of opportunity for early detection because progression from early to advanced cancer is slow.[5] However, being asymptomatic until an advanced stage, one-third of gastric cancers are metastatic at time of diagnosis.[5]

This article reviews the role of endoscopy, which is the modality of choice for the diagnosis of gastric cancer. Morphologic classification, the use adjunct technologies that aid in early detection and staging, and screening are also discussed.

CLASSIFICATION AND STAGING

Classification and staging of gastric cancer defines the disease and its behavior, dictates treatment decisions, and determines the prognosis. It also creates common grounds for communication among multiple care providers.

Gastric cancer is classified as early or advanced based on the distinct prognostic differences between these stages. Early gastric cancer (EGC) is limited to the gastric mucosa or submucosa irrespective of lymph node spread[6] and regardless of clinical presentation. EGC undergoes a period of slow growth with estimated median disease duration of 37 months before progression into advanced cancer.[7] In advanced cancer,

The authors have nothing to disclose.
[a] Division of Gastroenterology and Hepatology, University of Iowa Hospitals and Clinics, 200 Hawkins Drive, Iowa City, IA 52242, USA
[b] Diagnostic and Therapeutic Unit, Digestive Disease Center, University of Iowa Hospitals and Clinics, Iowa City, IA, USA
* Corresponding author.
E-mail address: rami-elabiad@uiowa.edu

tumor cells invade the muscularis propria and beyond. Patients with EGC tend to be younger and tend to have longer symptom duration.[8]

The International Union Against Cancer (UICC) and the American Joint Committee on Cancer (AJCC) use the tumor node metastasis (TNM) system for clinical (c) or pathologic (p) staging of gastric cancer. Proximal gastric tumors whose midpoint is at or within, 5 cm from the gastroesophageal junction follow TNM staging for esophageal adenocarcinoma. Tumors located further distally, in the fundus, body, and antrum of the stomach, follow the gastric TNM staging.

Depth of penetration of the primary tumor designates the T stage. The number of regional lymph nodes comprises the N stage, whereas distant (nonregional) lymph nodes, or peritoneal or other organ involvement, marks the M stage. EGC is a T1 category (**Table 1**).

The Lauren histologic classification into intestinal and diffuse types is traditionally used in the Western world.[9] The intestinal type, as the name implies, is characterized by the formation of glandular structures (intestinal metaplasia) comprising well-differentiated columnar epithelial cells. The diffuse type is characterized by pangastric

Table 1 TNM staging	
Primary Tumor (T)	
TX	Primary tumor cannot be assessed
T0	No evidence of primary tumor
Tis	Carcinoma in situ: intraepithelial tumor without invasion of the lamina propria
T1	Tumor invades lamina propria, muscularis mucosae, or submucosa
T1a	Tumor invades lamina propria or muscularis mucosae (T1m)
T1b	Tumor invades submucosa (T1sm)
T2	Tumor invades muscularis propria
T3	Tumor penetrates subserosal connective tissue without invasion of visceral peritoneum or adjacent structures
T4	Tumor invades serosa (visceral peritoneum) or adjacent structures
T4o	Tumor invades serosa (visceral peritoneum)
T4b	Tumor invades adjacent structures
Regional Lymph Nodes (N)	
NX	Regional lymph nodes cannot be assessed
N0	No regional lymph nodes
N1	Metastasis in 1–2 regional lymph nodes
N2	Metastasis in 3–6 regional lymph nodes
N3	Metastasis in 7 or more regional lymph nodes
N3a	Metastasis in 7–15 regional lymph nodes
NBb	Metastasis in 16 or more regional lymph nodes
Distant Metastasis	
M0	No distant metastasis
MI	Distant metastasis

Data from Washington K. 7th edition of the AJCC cancer staging manual: stomach. Ann Surg Oncol 2010;17:3077–9.

infiltration by poorly cohesive clusters or solitary mucin-rich (signet ring) cells. Transmural extension through lymphatic invasion can lead to gastric wall thickening without causing a discrete mass (linitis plastica).[9] Intestinal-type gastric cancer more commonly involves the distal stomach. It is closely linked to environmental (*Helicobacter pylori*) and dietary exposure and is declining. Diffuse-type gastric cancer tends to occur at a younger age and carries a worse prognosis.

Gastric cancer can exhibit different morphologic growth patterns. Advanced cancers are classified according to Borrmann (**Table 2**) into polypoid (type I) (**Fig. 1**), fungating (type II) (**Fig. 2**), ulcerated (type III) (**Fig. 3**), or infiltrative (type IV) (**Fig. 4**) cancers. The Paris endoscopic classification (**Table 3**) for superficial neoplastic lesions (type 0) incorporates the macroscopic classification system of the Japanese Gastric Cancer Association.[10] It distinguishes the polypoid type 0–I (subdivided into p, pedunculated; s, sessile), the superficial (or nonpolypoid) type 0–II (a, elevated [**Fig. 5**]; b, flat; c, depressed) and the excavated type 0–III (**Fig. 6**) with 0–IIa and 0–IIc being the most common variants.[11] Type 0–IIa lesions have a thickness equal to or less than twice that of the normal mucosa, whereas type 0–I lesions have a thickness that exceeds twice that of the normal mucosa. If a single lesion contains a combined pattern, the one occupying the greatest area is recorded first (**Fig. 7**).

ENDOSCOPIC DETECTION

Gastric cancer is usually asymptomatic until an advanced stage. If symptoms occur, they are similar to dyspepsia or peptic ulcer disease. Endoscopy is the procedure of choice for diagnosis. The accuracy of endoscopy in the detection and diagnosis of EGC is reported to range between 90% and 96%.[12] Endoscopy allows for tumor localization, morphologic characterization, and tissue diagnosis through biopsy. The American Gastroenterological Association recommends an upper endoscopy be performed in patients with new-onset dyspepsia who are older than 55 years as well as in patients with alarm symptoms (such as weight loss, recurrent vomiting, gastrointestinal [GI] bleeding, or family history of cancer).[13] The use of acid antisecretory therapy can mask symptoms and may delay early diagnosis.[14] EGC can assume different morphologic appearances on endoscopy, such as subtle polypoid protrusions, superficial

Table 2
The Borrmann classification of advanced gastric cancer

Type I		Polypoid tumors
Type II		Fungating carcinomas
Type III		Ulcerated carcinomas
Type IV		Infiltrating carcinomas

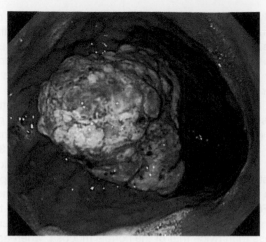

Fig. 1. Borrmann type I mass in the gastric body.

plaques, or depressions.[15] Ulcerated malignancies carry a higher risk of deep invasion and lymph node metastases compared with flat lesions.[16] The distinction between ulcerating cancer and benign peptic ulcers may not always be obvious[17] When a suspicious or nonhealing ulcer is encountered, 6 to 8 biopsy specimens from the edges and base of the ulcer are recommended. This number of specimens provides a 98% sensitivity to detect malignancy.[17,18] Brush cytology can add a little to the sensitivity.[19] Concerns about false-negative histology, which can approach 5%,[20] have been raised, and follow-up endoscopies have been advocated for all gastric ulcers to document healing.[21] However, studies revealed that endoscopic follow-up until complete healing yielded few malignancies and even fewer at early stages.[22,23] Because of the high sensitivity of multiple, adequately obtained biopsies, the usefulness of repeat endoscopy remains in question, especially if an experienced endoscopist deems the ulcer to be benign.

In the absence of a consensus, cautious practice is warranted in patients with gastric ulcers and increased pretest prevalence for gastric cancer. These high-risk patients include those with persistent upper GI symptoms despite adequate antisecretory therapy, those older than 50 years of age, those with family history of gastric cancer, or those who belong to certain ethnic groups in endemic areas (eg, Asians).

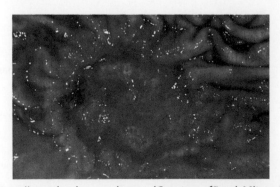

Fig. 2. Borrmann type II gastric adenocarcinoma. (*Courtesy of* Frank Mitros, MD, Iowa City, IA.)

A

B

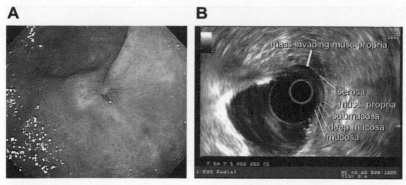

Fig. 3. (*A*) Small mass in the gastric antrum with thickened fold and focal depression (Borrmann type III). (*B*) Endoscopic ultrasonography (EUS) with a radial echoendoscope shows invasion into the muscularis propria (T2).

Absence of nonsteroidal antiinflammatory drug (NSAID) use should increase concern. Protracted history of peptic ulcer disease and concomitant presence of duodenal ulcers makes malignancy less likely.

The main method for discriminating malignant from benign ulcers is adequate biopsy. However, there are several criteria to macroscopically distinguish between benign and malignant ulcers based on endoscopic or radiologic findings. Benign gastric ulcers tend to have regular shapes (linear, round, or oval); even bases; smooth, sharply demarcated symmetric borders; and surrounding gastric folds that converge toward the ulcer.[24] Malignant gastric ulcers have geographic shapes; an uneven (sometimes shallow or necrotic) base; asymmetric elevated edges with rigid, thick, irregular borders; and disrupted periulcer folds near the crater edge and/or clubbed or fused folds.[25] Malignant ulcers may be associated with a mass lesion and the surrounding gastric mucosa may appear abnormal.[25] Although both benign and malignant ulcers can vary in size and can occur in multiplicity and in any location within the stomach, ulcers in the proximal half of the greater curvature and fundus should be

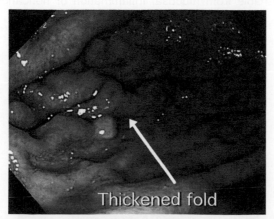

Fig. 4. Focal thickening of a gastric fold. This Borrmann type IV lesion represented cancer with invasion into the serosa (T4a). (*Courtesy of* Adrian Holm, DO, Iowa City, IA.)

Table 3
Paris classification of early gastric cancer (type 0)

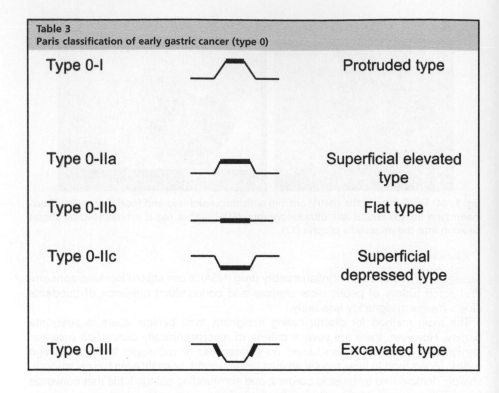

Type 0-I		Protruded type
Type 0-IIa		Superficial elevated type
Type 0-IIb		Flat type
Type 0-IIc		Superficial depressed type
Type 0-III		Excavated type

suspicious for malignancy.[26–29] Healed scars from benign gastric ulcers appear as collection of gastric folds converging toward a central pit.[26] An underlying malignancy should be suspected if the scar is irregular, has nodular edges, or the radiating folds are amputated.[26]

ENDOSCOPIC IMAGE–ENHANCING TECHNOLOGIES

EGC, which can appear as a flat lesion or superficial depression, can be endoscopically indistinguishable from mucosal inflammation or noncancerous erosions.

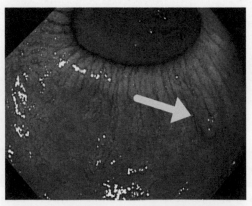

Fig. 5. Macroscopic type 0–IIa lesion (*arrow*). (*Courtesy of* Adrian Holm, DO, Iowa City, IA.)

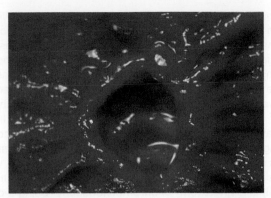

Fig. 6. Paris 0–III gastric adenocarcinoma. (*Courtesy of* Frank Mitros, MD, Iowa City, IA.)

Advancements in endoscope technologies improve the ability to detect and characterize gastric cancer. Additional image-enhancing methods and mucosal staining techniques are used to reduce the miss rate and to delineate margins facilitating endoscopic treatments such as endoscopic mucosal resection (EMR) and endoscopic submucosal dissection (ESD).

The introduction of high-definition endoscopes and the use of narrow-band imaging have yielded higher quality images with improved resolution and contrast. Magnification endoscopy, with its ability to evaluate fine mucosal surface patterns and microvasculature in real-time, may aid in the initial evaluation of lesions before histologic diagnosis. Endocytoscopy and confocal laser endomicroscopy, with 1000-fold magnification, permit in vivo high-resolution evaluation of the GI mucosa at the cellular

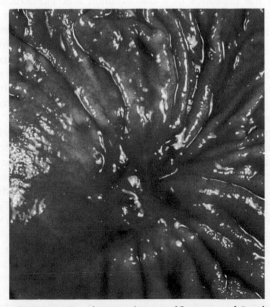

Fig. 7. Paris 0–IIc + 0–IIa gastric adenocarcinoma. (*Courtesy of* Frank Mitros, MD, Iowa City, IA.)

level, providing what has been termed optical biopsies.[30] Coupled with the instillation of chemicals such as acetic acid (enhanced magnification) or topical application of pigments or stains (magnification chromoendoscopy), the images can be further improved with visualization of fine surface patterns not seen with standard endoscopy. The following stains are commonly used to enhance mucosal contrast (chromoendoscopy): methylene blue (methylthionine chloride) is a carbon-based vital stain that selectively and reversibly binds to actively absorbing epithelium, such as gastric intestinal metaplasia,[31] and not to normal columnar gastric epithelium. Indigo carmine is a contrast stain that highlights fine mucosal morphology, aiding in recognition of subtle topographic changes. The instillation of acetic acid causes reversible alteration in tertiary structures of cellular proteins.[32] The acetic acid–induced whitening of the columnar mucosa produces an enhanced view of mucosal structures.[33,34] Narrowband imaging (NBI) is a virtual form of chromoendoscopy. Using a combination of 2 short wavelengths (415 nm and 540 nm) within a narrow bandwidth, NBI is capable of enhancing mucosal architecture and microvasculature.[35] Autofluorescence imaging videoendoscopy (AFI), which uses the autofluorescence of endogenous fluorophores (eg, collagen, nicotinamide, flavin, porphyrins, and adenine dinucleotide) from light excitation, produces real-time pseudocolor images[36] that can distinguish between (green) normal and dysplastic/neoplastic tissue (magenta purple).

These modalities, alone or in combination, have also been used in the identification of premalignant lesions within the intestinal-type gastric adenocarcinoma cascade (eg, intestinal metaplasia, dysplasia). However, most of the studies involving magnification endoscopy (enhanced or not) and chromoendoscopy that suggest improved discriminatory ability between benign, premalignant, and malignant lesions, remain descriptive.

Using magnification endoscopy (ME), Yao and colleagues[37] described 3 characteristic findings in differentiated gastric adenocarcinoma, including disappearance of regular subepithelial capillary network pattern, the presence of an irregular microvascular pattern, and the presence of a demarcation line. Nonstructural appearance caused by the lack of a normal tubular pattern suggests that the cancer involves the submucosal layer.[38] Tajiri and colleagues[39] described an irregular coarse mucosal surface pattern in elevated-type carcinomas and a finer pit pattern or destruction/disappearance of the mucosal microstructure and abnormal capillary vessels in depressed-type carcinomas. Otsuka and colleagues[40] classified the surface structure of EGC into small regular pattern of sulci and ridges, irregular pattern of sulci and ridges, or lack of visible structure. Microvasculature of cancerous lesions was described as either of varied caliber or minute and irregular.

With dynamic enhanced ME (EME), Yagi and colleagues[41] noticed that, compared with noncancerous gastric lesions, carcinomas returned faster to baseline color appearance after acetowhitening, further enhancing the margins between neoplastic and nonneoplastic tissue. Tanaka and colleagues,[42] using EME, described 5 surface patterns of gastric tumors and surrounding mucosa: small round pits of uniform size (type I), slitlike pits (type II), and fine villous or gyrus pattern (type III). Type IV is an irregular arrangement and sizes of the aforementioned patterns, and type V is a destructive pattern. All depressed-type EGCs were classified as type IV or V, whereas elevated-type cancers were classified as either type III or IV. The presence of types IV to V strongly correlated with underlying malignancy (sensitivity 100%, specificity 89.7%).[43]

ME-NBI is able to differentiate gastric tumors from background nonmalignant mucosa.[44] In a study of 136 patients, Dinis-Ribeiro and colleagues,[45] using magnification chromoendoscopy with methylene blue staining, classified gastric lesions based on mucosal and pit pattern with a diagnostic sensitivity and specificity of 76% and

87% respectively for intestinal metaplasia and 98% and 81% respectively for dysplasia. The reproducibility of this classification was further validated by Areia and colleagues.[46] Using ME-NBI, Sumiyama and colleagues[47] demarcated EGC based on differences in capillary structures. Kato and colleagues[48] showed that, in patients who had lesions previously identified with white-light endoscopy (WLE), ME-NBI is superior to WLE in diagnosis of gastric cancer when the diagnostic triad of the disappearance of fine mucosal structure, microvascular dilation, and heterogeneity is used. Triad-based diagnosis by ME-NBI had sensitivity and specificity of 92.9% and 94.7% respectively, compared with 43% sensitivity and 61% specificity of WLE. In a prospective study involving 57 gastric depressive lesions smaller than 10 mm, Ezoe and colleagues[49] found that the diagnostic accuracy was significantly better for ME-NBI than for ME using white-light imaging (79% vs 44%) as was the sensitivity (70% vs 33%), with no significant difference in specificity. Kadowaki and colleagues[50] compared 4 methods of ME: conventional ME (CME), EME, ME-NBI, and EME-NBI. Despite the small number of enrolled patients (n = 37) EME-NBI was significantly better than CME alone in identifying EGC demarcation, followed by EME or ME-NBI.

Kiyotoki and colleagues[51] found ME-NBI to be significantly more accurate than indigo carmine chromoendoscopy (97% vs 78% respectively) in identifying tumor margins in patients undergoing ESD for EGC.

ENDOSCOPIC ULTRASOUND

Because distinct wall layers of the luminal GI tract can be visualized with endoscopic ultrasound (EUS), the technique is used to assess the penetration depth of GI malignancies and hence determine the T category according to the TNM classification. In addition, EUS can be used to assess locoregional lymphadenopathy and involvement of adjacent organs. EUS can be accomplished with dedicated echoendoscopes with built-in linear or radial ultrasound transducers or with ultrasound catheter probes that are passed through the accessory channel of a gastroscope. Depending on the frequencies that are used, 5 to 9 layers of the gastric wall can be distinguished by EUS based on their alternating bright (hyperechoic) and dark (hypoechoic) appearance. Through-the-scope ultrasound probes with high frequencies (12–20 MHz) provide high-resolution images of small superficial lesions at the cost of limited field of view and penetration depth. Conversely, echoendoscopes operate at frequencies from 5 to 12 MHz and are more suitable for larger lesions, assessment of lymph node metastases, and invasion of adjacent organs. Linear-array echoendoscopes can be used to obtain EUS-guided biopsies if tissue confirmation is required for suspected metastases.

EUS has not been as widely adopted for the staging of gastric cancer as for rectal and esophageal cancer. However, there is increasing interest in precise preoperative staging of gastric cancer with individualized treatment protocols that include neoadjuvant regimens for advanced cancers and curative endoscopic resection of superficial cancers.

T STAGE

A recent meta-analysis of 54 clinical studies found that EUS distinguishes T1 to T2 cancer from T3 to T4 cancer with a sensitivity of 86% and a specificity of 91%.[52] Classification of specific T categories was less accurate, and there was significant heterogeneity among studies. Included studies used former versions of the TNM system. With recent modification of T categories, invasion of the subserosa, formerly T2b, is classified as T3, and penetration of the serosa, formerly T3, is now T4a.[53] Hence, distinction between T1 to T2 and T3 to T4 translates into distinction between T1 to T3 and T4 with the updated classification. The new definitions may make accurate EUS classification of T2 to T4a more difficult. The distinction of subserosa from serosa may be impossible with EUS and further difficulty arises from parts of the stomach, such as the posterior fundus and lesser curvature, not possessing a serosa. Previous concerns of overstaging T2 as T3 using the former TNM system[54,55] now shift to over-staging T3 as T4a. Likewise, invasion into the subserosa may be difficult to detect with EUS if the outer tumor margin remains smooth, which may result in understaging T3 (subserosal invasion) as T2 (not beyond muscularis propria). Thus, overstaging and understaging is most likely to occur in patients with true T3 cancers. Studies evaluating the impact of the revised T categories on EUS staging accuracy and clinical decision making are not yet available.

N STAGE

In contrast with the high reported accuracy regarding the T category, EUS is less reliable for the assessment of nodal involvement. Sensitivity and specificity for lymph node involvement were 69% and 84% in the recent meta-analysis.[52] Endosonographic criteria for malignant lymph nodes include sharp contour, round shape, hypoechoic echo pattern, and large size (>10 mm). Confirmation of lymph node metastases through EUS-guided biopsies may be helpful in some cases.

COMPARISON WITH OTHER IMAGING MODALITIES

Compared with computed tomography (CT), EUS has been reported to be superior in T staging.[56] However, with recent technical advances including multidetector CT (MDCT) and three-dimensional (3D) reconstruction, the performance of CT for T staging is close to that of EUS.[57,58] A systematic review published in 2007 that included 22 EUS studies, 5 MDCT studies, 1 combined EUS and MDCT study, and 3 magnetic resonance imaging (MRI) studies found similar accuracies of these imaging modalities for T staging and serosal invasion.[59] Reported accuracies of nodal staging with EUS, CT, MRI, and positron emission tomography are variable and not consistently high with any of these modalities.[60]

METASTATIC DISEASE

EUS is not usually relied on to exclude distant metastases although, in a prospective study comparing linear-array EUS with CT, there was a trend in favor of EUS to detect liver metastases.[61] Contrary to popular belief, the right lobe of the liver can be visualized with EUS and is accessible for EUS-guided fine-needle aspiration. EUS with fine-needle aspiration is also useful for lesions that are too small to be characterized by CT. However, the entire liver cannot be seen in every patient and especially subdiaphragmatic portions of the right lobe may not be visualized. It is the authors' opinion that the liver is best examined with a curved-linear echoendoscope both from the stomach and from the duodenal bulb.

In a retrospective study, EUS with fine-needle aspiration for suspected distant metastases changed the management from surgical resection to palliative treatment in 15% of patients who underwent EUS.[62] However, a large proportion of cases with metastatic disease were adenocarcinomas of the gastric cardia with metastases to mediastinal lymph nodes. Most cancers in this location meet the current definition of gastroesophageal junction tumors if they are located within 5 cm of the gastroesophageal junction.[53] For these, mediastinal lymph nodes are regarded as locoregional. Nevertheless, the authors have also found hepatic metastases that were not seen by CT, mediastinal lymph node metastases in cancers of the gastric body and antrum, an adrenal gland metastasis, and malignant ascites.

EUS can detect even trace amounts of ascites. This finding is highly predictive of peritoneal metastases in patients with gastric cancer.[63] In a prospective study, the ability to diagnose peritoneal metastases through detection of ascites with EUS was comparable with surgical staging through laparoscopy and laparotomy.[63] In contrast, another series found that macroscopic peritoneal carcinomatosis was only seen in 14% of patients with ascites on EUS, resulting in a low specificity of this finding.[54] This study was criticized for its retrospective design and the diagnosis of peritoneal metastases only being based on macroscopic carcinomatosis and not including cytology of peritoneal lavage fluid. In another study that was prospectively conducted with ultrasound catheter probes, the finding of ascites was highly specific for peritoneal seeding but the sensitivity was low (61%), which could be because of the limited ultrasound penetration of the catheter probes compared with conventional echoendoscopes.[64] A systematic review that included 4 EUS studies found that EUS is superior to CT and transabdominal ultrasound in diagnosing peritoneal metastases but not reliable enough to replace preoperative laparoscopy.[65] It has been suggested that EUS is helpful to select patients who benefit from laparoscopy because the yield of laparoscopy to detect metastatic disease is low unless high-risk criteria are found by EUS (>T2 or N1).[66]

EUS FOR EGC

EGC may be amenable for EMR or ESD. Invasion of the muscularis propria (T2) is a clear contraindication for endoscopic resection and needs to be excluded. As confirmed by a recent meta-analysis,[52] EUS can distinguish early cancer (T1) from more advanced cancer with good sensitivity (83%) and excellent specificity (96%). A greater challenge is the distinction between cancers confined to the mucosa (T1a) and those with submucosal invasion (T1b). This distinction is clinically important because submucosal invasion increases the risk of lymph node metastasis and usually precludes a curative endoscopic approach. However, it has been proposed to expand the indication for endoscopic resection to cancer with minimal submucosa invasion (<500 μm) if certain low-risk criteria are met.[67] Thus, it is important to distinguish early cancer with mucosal, minimal submucosal, and deep submucosal invasion. In this context, high-frequency ultrasound probes have the advantage of providing finer visualization of the gastric wall layers than conventional echoendoscopes that operate with lower ultrasound frequencies. Reported results of EUS have been heterogeneous. In a systematic review that included 18 studies, sensitivities and specificities for invasion beyond the mucosa ranged from 18.2% to 100% (median 87.8%) and from 34.7% to 100% (median 80.2%), respectively.[68] Sensitivities were more homogeneous in 8 studies that used ultrasound frequencies of 15 MHz or higher (pooled sensitivity 87%) and studies that exclusively included patients who were endoscopically suspected of having early gastric cancer (pooled sensitivity 91%). Specificities remained heterogeneous in these subgroups. In a large recent study, EUS with high-frequency catheter probes correctly identified a combined group of mucosal and superficial submucosal invasion in 81%.[69] Factors that lower the accuracy of EUS are large cancer diameter (>3 cm), ulceration, undifferentiated histology, and proximal location.[69–71] Based on these reported performance characteristic, EUS, especially if performed with high-frequency catheters by experienced experts, seems to be helpful in selecting patients for endoscopic resection. However, assessment with standard endoscopy alone may enable accurate prediction of the invasion depth.[72] Skepticism regarding the role of EUS is nurtured by 2 studies that did not find EUS to be more accurate than standard endoscopy in predicting submucosal invasion.[70,73] Endoscopic criteria for submucosal invasion include an uneven base, irregularly shaped nodules, and enlarged folds.[73] Standard endoscopy tends to understage lesions with submucosal invasion, whereas EUS tends to overstage mucosal lesions because of benign reactive submucosal changes.[73]

LINITIS PLASTICA

In linitis plastica (**Fig. 8**D), the diffusely infiltrating tumor triggers a desmoplastic response rendering the stomach stiff.[74] Grossly, the stomach appears thickened with shrunken lumen resembling a leather bottle on contrast imaging (see **Fig. 8**A, B).[75] On endoscopic examination, linitis plastica is characterized by thickened gastric folds, impaired distensibility of the involved portion of the stomach, and a distinct boundary toward the uninvolved stomach. Peristalsis may also be abnormal. However, there may be no, or only mild, nonspecific mucosal surface changes unless the cancer breaks through the mucosa and creates ulcers or erosions. The typical EUS appearance of linitis plastica is diffuse hypoechoic wall thickening with disruption of the wall architecture (see **Fig. 8**C). Histologic confirmation of the diagnosis can be challenging because endoscopic surface biopsies are frequently nondiagnostic.[76] In these cases, a diagnosis may be achieved through tunnel biopsies (sampling the same area

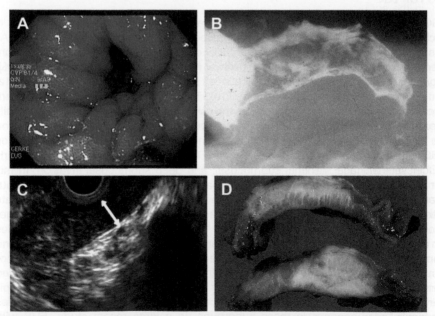

Fig. 8. (*A*) Endoscopic appearance of thickened folds in the gastric antrum with lack of distensibility. (*B*) Double-contrast upper gastrointestinal study of scirrhous carcinoma revealing thickened gastric wall and poor distensibility. (*C*) EUS with a linear-curved-array echoendoscope shows diffuse hypoechoic gastric wall thickening (*arrow*) with loss of the layered architecture. (*D*) Pathologic appearance of linitis plastica with diffuse gastric wall thickening caused by tumor infiltration and secondary desmoplastic response.

repetitively with large biopsy forceps to get into deeper tissue layers), snare biopsies, or mucosal resection. EUS-guided core biopsies of the gastric wall using an EUS Trucut needle may also be helpful.[77] However, negative biopsies do not exclude malignancy, and surgical exploration may be required in the presence of typical endoscopic and endosonographic findings.

Unexplained gastric wall thickening on CT is a common indication for endoscopic evaluation. This finding is nonspecific and the yield of EUS is low if standard endoscopy shows no mucosal changes and normal gastric distensibility.[78]

SCREENING

Gastric cancer screening for asymptomatic individuals remains controversial.[79] Screening methods vary in different settings but the effectiveness of each remains unsettled.[80,81] Mass screening programs have been implemented in areas of high disease incidence. Since the 1960s, Japan has used a gastric cancer screening program in which individuals older than 40 years undergo double-contrast barium study followed by an upper endoscopy if any abnormality is detected. Serum pepsinogen tests have been used to select patients for screening endoscopies because they identify patients who are at increased risk for extensive atrophic gastritis.[82] A systematic review, commissioned by the Japanese Ministry of Health, evaluated barium radiograph study, endoscopy, serum pepsinogen testing, and H pylori antibody testing as screening modalities for gastric cancer.[83,84] Barium radiograph studies carried the highest level of evidence for cancer detection (sensitivity of 60%–80% and specificity of 80%–90%) and mortality reduction (5-year survival rates of 74%–80% in the screened group vs 46%–56% in the unscreened group). In the limited available studies, the sensitivity of endoscopy was 78%, with no reported data on specificity. The effect of upper endoscopy on survival benefit was not available. The sensitivity of serum pepsinogen test decreased in the 40% to 80% range, with specificity less than 80%. The sensitivity of H pylori antibody testing was 88%, with specificity as low as 41%. These data were part of the analytical framework leading to the institution of barium radiograph as the initial study of choice for population-based and opportunistic screening for gastric cancer in Japan. Although mass screening programs from Japan are generally considered to be effective,[85] there remains a question as to whether detection of EGC translates into survival benefits. The cost-effectiveness also depends on the incidence of gastric cancer. In a high-risk group of Chinese men (age standardized incidence of 25.9 per 100,000 population) the cost of endoscopic screening was found to be $28,836 per quality-adjusted life years saved, almost 10 times cheaper than the cost of averting 1 gastric cancer death in men in the United States (assuming an incidence of gastric cancer less than 10 per 100,000 population).[86]

In areas of low incidence, case finding, which involves screening a smaller group of people based on the presence of risk factors, is thought to be more appropriate.[87] Populations at increased risk include patients with atrophic gastritis or pernicious anemia,[88] patients after partial gastrectomy,[89] patients with a sporadic gastric adenoma,[90] ethnic groups that immigrated from areas of high incidence, and patients with familial adenomatous polyposis (FAP) and hereditary nonpolyposis colon cancer (HNPCC).[4,91] The American Society for Gastrointestinal Endoscopy (ASGE) published updated guidelines in 2006[92] for endoscopic screening and surveillance that, in most parts, leave the endoscopist free to select a reasonable interval by individualizing follow-up. One-year repeat esophagogastroduodenostomy (EGD) is recommended after polypectomy of gastric adenoma to assess for recurrence and to rule out metachronous polyps. If negative, then 3-year to 5-year surveillance intervals are suggested. In patients with gastric intestinal metaplasia, the issue of surveillance remains unsettled. Short surveillance intervals, as frequent as every 3 months, versus intervention have been proposed in the presence of dysplasia. Although routine surveillance in patients with pernicious anemia lacks supportive data, a single endoscopy soon after the diagnosis is suggested to identify precancerous lesions. This endoscopy may be followed by further individualized surveillance based on the findings at index endoscopy. After partial gastric resection for peptic ulcer disease, surveillance endoscopy should be considered within 15 to 20 years. In patients with FAP syndrome, upper endoscopy could be performed at the time of colectomy or in the third decade of life. Repeat examination should be obtained in 5 years if no adenomas were detected. Similarly, in patients with Lynch syndrome (HNPCC), EGD at age 30 years might be beneficial, but surveillance interval remains uncertain. Until the natural history of gastric carcinogenesis is completely understood, the available uncontrolled studies that suggest reduction in mortality with screening[93-96] may prove to be inadequate when lead time bias, length time bias, and selection bias are considered.

SUMMARY

Gastric cancer is a common disease with significant medical burden. Endoscopy with adequate biopsies is the gold standard for diagnosis. Missed lesions remain a concern, especially in early disease in which the chances of cure are high. The advancement of technology in endoscopy and radiologic imaging has added to the armamentarium for early diagnosis and staging. However, clinicians must be aware of the limitations of these modalities and the role of each has to be further refined. Screening patients in areas of high disease incidence, or those with risk factors, may be of benefit.

ACKNOWLEDGMENTS

We wish to thank Frank Mitros, MD, Department of Pathology, and Adrian Holm, DO, Division of Gastroenterology and Hepatology, University of Iowa Hospitals and Clinics, Iowa City, Iowa, for their contribution to the images.

REFERENCES

1. Available at: http://globocan.iarc.fr/factsheets/cancers/stomach.asp. Accessed May 1, 2011.
2. Available at: http://www.who.int/mediacentre/factsheets/fs297/en/index.html. Accessed May 1, 2011.
3. Available at: http://seer.cancer.gov/csr/1975_2008/results_merged/sect_24_stomach.pdf. Accessed May 1, 2011.
4. Alexander JR, Andrews JM, Buchi KN, et al. High prevalence of adenomatous polyps of the duodenal papilla in familial adenomatous polyposis. Dig Dis Sci 1989;34(2):167-70.
5. Jemal A, Siegel R, Ward E, et al. Cancer statistics, 2007. CA Cancer J Clin 2007; 57(1):43-66.
6. Murakami T. Pathomorphological diagnosis. Definition and gross classification of early gastric cancer. Gann Monogr Cancer Res 1971;11:53.
7. Tsukuma H, Mishima T, Oshima A. Prospective study of "early" gastric cancer. Int J Cancer 1983;31(4):421-6.

8. Eckardt VF, Giessler W, Kanzler G, et al. Clinical and morphological characteristics of early gastric cancer. A case-control study. Gastroenterology 1990;98(3): 708–14.

9. Lauren P. The two histological main types of gastric carcinoma: diffuse and so-called intestinal-type carcinoma. An attempt at a histo-clinical classification. Acta Pathol Microbiol Scand 1965;64:31–49.

10. Japanese Gastric Cancer Association. Japanese classification of gastric carcinoma - 2nd English edition. Gastric Cancer 1998;1:10–24.

11. The Paris endoscopic classification of superficial neoplastic lesions: esophagus, stomach, and colon: November 30 to December 1, 2002. Gastrointest Endosc 2003;58(Suppl 6):S3–43.

12. Ballantyne KC, Morris DL, Jones JA, et al. Accuracy of identification of early gastric cancer. Br J Surg 1987;74(7):618–9.

13. Talley NJ, American Gastroenterological Association. American Gastroenterological Association medical position statement: evaluation of dyspepsia. Gastroenterology 2005;129(5):1753–5.

14. Suvakovic Z, Bramble MG, Jones R, et al. Improving the detection rate of early gastric cancer requires more than open access gastroscopy: a five year study. Gut 1997;41(3):308–13.

15. Kajitani T. The general rules for the gastric cancer study in surgery and pathology. Part I. Clinical classification. Jpn J Surg 1981;11(2):127–39.

16. Torii A, Sakai M, Inoue K, et al. A clinicopathological analysis of early gastric cancer: retrospective study with special reference to lymph node metastasis. Cancer Detect Prev 1994;18(6):437–41.

17. Graham DY, Schwartz JT, Cain GD, et al. Prospective evaluation of biopsy number in the diagnosis of esophageal and gastric carcinoma. Gastroenterology 1982;82(2):228–31.

18. Farley DR, Donohue JH. Early gastric cancer. Surg Clin N Am 1992;72(2):401–21.

19. Wang HH, Jonasson JG, Ducatman BS, et al. Brushing cytology of the upper gastrointestinal tract. Obsolete or not? Acta Cytol 1991;35(2):195–8.

20. Llanos O, Guzman S, Duarte I. Accuracy of the first endoscopic procedure in the differential diagnosis of gastric lesions. Ann Surg 1982;195(2):224–6.

21. Saini SD, Eisen G, Mattek N, et al. Utilization of upper endoscopy for surveillance of gastric ulcers in the United States. Am J Gastroenterol 2008;103(8): 1920–5.

22. Malmaeus J, Nilsson F. Endoscopy in the management of gastric ulcer disease. Acta Chir Scand 1981;147(7):551–3.

23. Trägårdh B, Haglund U. Endoscopic diagnosis of gastric ulcer. Evaluation of the benefits of endoscopic follow-up observation for malignancy. Acta Chir Scand 1985;151(1):37–41.

24. Eisenberg RL. Gastric ulcers. Gastrointestinal radiology: a pattern approach. Philadelphia: Lippincott Williams & Wilkins; 2003. p. 181.

25. Maruyama M, Baba Y. Gastric carcinoma. Radiol Clin N Am 1994;32(6):1233–52.

26. Gore RM, Levine MS, Ghahremani GG, et al. Gastric cancer. Radiologic diagnosis. Radiol Clin N Am 1997;35(2):311–29.

27. Taxin RN, Livingston PA, Seaman WB. Multiple gastric ulcers: a radiographic sign of benignity? Radiology 1975;114(1):23–7.

28. Dupont BJ Jr, Cohn I Jr. Gastric adenocarcinoma. Curr Probl Cancer 1980;4(8): 1–46.

29. Findley Jw JR. Ulcers of the greater curvature of the stomach. Gastroenterology 1961;40:183–7.

30. Inoue H, Kazawa T, Sato Y, et al. In vivo observation of living cancer cells in the esophagus, stomach, and colon using catheter-type contact endoscope, "Endo-Cytoscopy system". Gastrointest Endosc Clin N Am 2004;14(3): 589–94.
31. Morales TG, Bhattacharyya A, Camargo E, et al. Methylene blue staining for intestinal metaplasia of the gastric cardia with follow-up for dysplasia. Gastrointest Endosc 1998;48(1):26–31.
32. Lambert R, Rey JF, Sankaranarayanan R. Magnification and chromoscopy with the acetic acid test. Endoscopy 2003;35(5):437–45.
33. Guelrud M, Herrera I, Essenfeld H, et al. Enhanced magnification endoscopy: a new technique to identify specialized intestinal metaplasia in Barrett's esophagus. Gastrointest Endosc 2001;53(6):559–65.
34. Guelrud M, Herrera I, Essenfeld H, et al. Intestinal metaplasia of the gastric cardia: a prospective study with enhanced magnification endoscopy. Am J Gastroenterol 2002;97(3):584–9.
35. Gono K, Yamazaki K, Doguchi N, et al. Endoscopic observation of tissue by narrow-band illumination. Opt Rev 2003;10:1–5.
36. Haringsma J, Tytgat GN, Yano H, et al. Autofluorescence endoscopy: feasibility of detection of GI neoplasms unapparent to white light endoscopy with an evolving technology. Gastrointest Endosc 2001;53(6):642–50.
37. Yao K, Iwashita A, Yao T. Early gastric cancer: proposal for a new diagnostic system based on microvascular architecture as visualized by magnified endoscopy. Dig Endosc 2004;16(Suppl):S110–7.
38. Yoshida T, Kawachi H, Sasajima K, et al. The clinical meaning of a nonstructural pattern in early gastric cancer on magnifying endoscopy. Gastrointest Endosc 2005;62(1):48–54.
39. Tajiri H, Doi T, Endo H, et al. Routine endoscopy using a magnifying endoscope for gastric cancer diagnosis. Endoscopy 2002;34(10):772–7.
40. Otsuka Y, Niwa Y, Ohmiya N, et al. Usefulness of magnifying endoscopy in the diagnosis of early gastric cancer. Endoscopy 2004;36(2):165–9.
41. Yagi K, Aruga Y, Nakamura A, et al. The study of dynamic chemical magnifying endoscopy in gastric neoplasia. Gastrointest Endosc 2005;62(6):963–9.
42. Tanaka K, Toyoda H, Hamada Y, et al. Endoscopic submucosal dissection for early gastric cancer using magnifying endoscopy with a combination of narrow imaging and acetic acid instillation. Dig Endosc 2008;20:150–3.
43. Tanaka K, Toyoda H, Kadowaki S, et al. Surface pattern classification by enhanced-magnification endoscopy for identifying early gastric cancers. Gastrointest Endosc 2008;67(3):430–7.
44. Uedo N, Ishihara R, Iishi H, et al. A new method of diagnosing gastric intestinal metaplasia: narrow-band imaging with magnifying endoscopy. Endoscopy 2006; 38(8):819–24.
45. Dinis-Ribeiro M, da Costa-Pereira A, Lopes C, et al. Magnification chromoendoscopy for the diagnosis of gastric intestinal metaplasia and dysplasia. Gastrointest Endosc 2003;57(4):498–504.
46. Areia M, Amaro P, Dinis-Ribeiro M, et al. External validation of a classification for methylene blue magnification chromoendoscopy in premalignant gastric lesions. Gastrointest Endosc 2008;67(7):1011–8.
47. Sumiyama K, Kaise M, Nakayoshi T, et al. Combined use of a magnifying endoscope with a narrow band imaging system and a multibending endoscope for en bloc EMR of early stage gastric cancer. Gastrointest Endosc 2004;60(1):79–84.

48. Kato M, Kaise M, Yonezawa J, et al. Magnifying endoscopy with narrow-band imaging achieves superior accuracy in the differential diagnosis of superficial gastric lesions identified with white-light endoscopy: a prospective study. Gastrointest Endosc 2010;72(3):523–9.

49. Ezoe Y, Muto M, Horimatsu T, et al. Magnifying narrow-band imaging versus magnifying white-light imaging for the differential diagnosis of gastric small depressive lesions: a prospective study. Gastrointest Endosc 2010;71(3): 477–84.

50. Kadowaki S, Tanaka K, Toyoda H, et al. Ease of early gastric cancer demarcation recognition: a comparison of four magnifying endoscopy methods. J Gastroenterol Hepatol 2009;24(10):1625–30.

51. Kiyotoki S, Nishikawa J, Satake M, et al. Usefulness of magnifying endoscopy with narrow-band imaging for determining gastric tumor margin. J Gastroenterol Hepatol 2010;25(10):1636–41.

52. Mocellin S, Marchet A, Nitti D. EUS for the staging of gastric cancer: a meta-analysis. Gastrointest Endosc 2011;73:1122–34.

53. Washington K. 7th edition of the AJCC cancer staging manual: stomach. Ann Surg Oncol 2010;17:3077–9.

54. Chen CH, Yang CC, Yeh YH. Preoperative staging of gastric cancer by endoscopic ultrasound: the prognostic usefulness of ascites detected by endoscopic ultrasound. J Clin Gastroenterol 2002;35:321–7.

55. Shimoyama S, Yasuda H, Hashimoto M, et al. Accuracy of linear-array EUS for preoperative staging of gastric cardia cancer. Gastrointest Endosc 2004;60: 50–5.

56. Polkowski M, Palucki J, Wronska E, et al. Endosonography versus helical computed tomography for locoregional staging of gastric cancer. Endoscopy 2004;36:617–23.

57. Bhandari S, Shim CS, Kim JH, et al. Usefulness of three-dimensional, multidetector row CT (virtual gastroscopy and multiplanar reconstruction) in the evaluation of gastric cancer: a comparison with conventional endoscopy, EUS, and histopathology. Gastrointest Endosc 2004;59:619–26.

58. Hwang SW, Lee DH, Lee SH, et al. Preoperative staging of gastric cancer by endoscopic ultrasonography and multidetector-row computed tomography. J Gastroenterol Hepatol 2010;25:512–8.

59. Kwee RM, Kwee TC. Imaging in local staging of gastric cancer: a systematic review. J Clin Oncol 2007;25:2107–16.

60. Kwee RM, Kwee TC. Imaging in assessing lymph node status in gastric cancer. Gastric Cancer 2009;12:6–22.

61. Singh P, Mukhopadhyay P, Bhatt B, et al. Endoscopic ultrasound versus CT scan for detection of the metastases to the liver: results of a prospective comparative study. J Clin Gastroenterol 2009;43:367–73.

62. Hassan H, Vilmann P, Sharma V. Impact of EUS-guided FNA on management of gastric carcinoma. Gastrointest Endosc 2010;71:500–4.

63. Lee YT, Ng EK, Hung LC, et al. Accuracy of endoscopic ultrasonography in diagnosing ascites and predicting peritoneal metastases in gastric cancer patients. Gut 2005;54:1541–5.

64. Chu KM, Kwok KF, Law S, et al. A prospective evaluation of catheter probe EUS for the detection of ascites in patients with gastric carcinoma. Gastrointest Endosc 2004;59:471–4.

65. Wang Z, Chen JQ. Imaging in assessing hepatic and peritoneal metastases of gastric cancer: a systematic review. BMC Gastroenterol 2011;11:19.

66. Power DG, Schattner MA, Gerdes H, et al. Endoscopic ultrasound can improve the selection for laparoscopy in patients with localized gastric cancer. J Am Coll Surg 2009;208:173–8.
67. Soetikno R, Kaltenbach T, Yeh R, et al. Endoscopic mucosal resection for early cancers of the upper gastrointestinal tract. J Clin Oncol 2005;23:4490–8.
68. Kwee RM, Kwee TC. The accuracy of endoscopic ultrasonography in differentiating mucosal from deeper gastric cancer. Am J Gastroenterol 2008;103:1801–9.
69. Okada K, Fujisaki J, Kasuga A, et al. Endoscopic ultrasonography is valuable for identifying early gastric cancers meeting expanded-indication criteria for endoscopic submucosal dissection. Surg Endosc 2011;25:841–8.
70. Choi J, Kim SG, Im JP, et al. Comparison of endoscopic ultrasonography and conventional endoscopy for prediction of depth of tumor invasion in early gastric cancer. Endoscopy 2010;42:705–13.
71. Tsuzuki T, Okada H, Kawahara Y, et al. Usefulness and problems of endoscopic ultrasonography in prediction of the depth of tumor invasion in early gastric cancer. Acta Med Okayama 2011;65:105–12.
72. Choi J, Kim SG, Im JP, et al. Endoscopic prediction of tumor invasion depth in early gastric cancer. Gastrointest Endosc 2011;73:917–27.
73. Yanai H, Matsumoto Y, Harada T, et al. Endoscopic ultrasonography and endoscopy for staging depth of invasion in early gastric cancer: a pilot study. Gastrointest Endosc 1997;46:212–6.
74. Levine MS, Kong V, Rubesin SE, et al. Scirrhous carcinoma of the stomach: radiologic and endoscopic diagnosis. Radiology 1990;175(1):151–4.
75. Balthazar EJ, Rosenberg H, Davidian MM. Scirrhous carcinoma of the pyloric channel and distal antrum. AJR Am J Roentgenol 1980;134(4):669–73.
76. Andriulli A, Recchia S, De Angelis C, et al. Endoscopic ultrasonographic evaluation of patients with biopsy negative gastric linitis plastica. Gastrointest Endosc 1990;36:611–5.
77. Thomas T, Kaye PV, Ragunath K, et al. Endoscopic-ultrasound-guided mural trucut biopsy in the investigation of unexplained thickening of esophagogastric wall. Endoscopy 2009;41:335–9.
78. Lam EC, Rego RR, Paquin SC, et al. In patients referred for investigation because computed tomography suggests thickened gastric folds, endoscopic ultrasound is superfluous if gastroscopy is normal. Am J Gastroenterol 2007;102:1200–3.
79. Leung WK, Wu MS, Kakugawa Y, et al. Screening for gastric cancer in Asia: current evidence and practice. Lancet Oncol 2008;9(3):279–87.
80. Mizoue T, Yoshimura T, Tokui N, et al. Prospective study of screening for stomach cancer in Japan. Int J Cancer 2003;106(1):103–7.
81. Pisani P, Oliver WE, Parkin DM, et al. Case-control study of gastric cancer screening in Venezuela. Br J Cancer 1994;69(6):1102–5.
82. Miki K. Gastric cancer screening using the serum pepsinogen test method. Gastric Cancer 2006;9(4):245–53.
83. Hamashima C, Shibuya D, Yamazaki H, et al. The Japanese guidelines for gastric cancer screening. Jpn J Clin Oncol 2008;38(4):259–67.
84. Hamashima C, Saito H, Nakayama T, et al. The standardized development method of the Japanese guidelines for cancer screening. Jpn J Clin Oncol 2008;38(4):288–95.
85. Murakami R, Tsukuma H, Ubukata T, et al. Estimation of validity of mass screening program for gastric cancer in Osaka, Japan. Cancer 1990;65(5):1255–60.
86. Dan YY, So JB, Yeoh KG. Endoscopic screening for gastric cancer. Clin Gastroenterol Hepatol 2006;4(6):709–16.

87. Sackett DL, Holland WW. Controversy in the detection of disease. Lancet 1975; 2(7930):357–9.
88. Kokkola A, Sjoblom SM, Haapiainen R, et al. The risk of gastric carcinoma and carcinoid tumours in patients with pernicious anaemia. A prospective follow-up study. Scand J Gastroenterol 1998;33(1):88–92.
89. Lundegårdh G, Adami HO, Helmick C, et al. Stomach cancer after partial gastrectomy for benign ulcer disease. N Engl J Med 1988;319(4):195–200.
90. Ming SC, Goldman H. Gastric Polyps; a histogenetic classification and its relation to carcinoma. Cancer 1965;18:721–6.
91. Aarnio M, Salovaara R, Aaltonen LA, et al. Features of gastric cancer in hereditary non-polyposis colorectal cancer syndrome. Int J Cancer 1997;74(5):551–5.
92. Hirota WK, Zuckerman MJ, Adler DG, et al. ASGE guideline: the role of endoscopy in the surveillance of premalignant conditions of the upper GI tract. Gastrointest Endosc 2006;63(4):570–80.
93. Hisamichi S, Sugawara N, Fukao A. Effectiveness of gastric mass screening in Japan. Cancer Detect Prev 1988;11:323–9.
94. Fukao A, Tsubono Y, Tsuji I, et al. The evaluation of screening for gastric cancer in Miyagi Prefecture, Japan: a population-based case-control study. Int J Cancer 1995;60(1):45–8.
95. Kunisaki C, Ishino J, Nakajima S, et al. Outcomes of mass screening for gastric carcinoma. Ann Surg Oncol 2006;13(2):221–8.
96. Oshima A, Hirata N, Ubukata T, et al. Evaluation of a mass screening program for stomach cancer with a case-control study design. Int J Cancer 1986;38(6): 829–33.

Gastrointestinal Stromal Tumors of the Stomach

Joseph J. Bennett, MD*, Matthew S. Rubino, MD

KEYWORDS

- Gastrointestinal stromal tumor • Tyrosine kinase inhibitor
- GIST • Imatinib • Sunitinib

Gastrointestinal stromal tumors (GISTs) are mesenchymal tumors that are thought to be derived from the interstitial cells of Cajal within the gastrointestinal tract.[1,2] GISTs can occur anywhere along the gastrointestinal tract, from the esophagus to the rectum. The most common primary site is the stomach (50%), followed by the small intestine (36%), colon (7%), rectum (5%), and esophagus (1%).[3]

Recent estimates place the incidence of GISTs at between 5,000[4] and 10,000[5] cases per year in the United States. Tran and colleagues[3] conducted a population-based analysis of the Surveillance Epidemiology and End Results (SEER) database, including 1,458 patients with GISTs between 1992 and 2000. They found a yearly incidence of 0.68 per 100,000 during the study period. They also found a 1.5-fold higher incidence of GISTs in men (0.83/100,000) than in women (0.57/100,000). There was a higher incidence of GISTs in blacks (1.16/100,000) than in other races (0.97/100,000), with the lowest incidence in whites (0.60/100,000). The mean age of diagnosis was 62.9 years and the incidence increased with age. The impact of the anatomic location of GISTs on overall survival has been controversial in the literature. Some studies have suggested that gastric GISTs are less aggressive than GISTs of the lower gastrointestinal tract,[6] whereas others suggest no difference.[7] In this large SEER database study, the anatomic location had no impact on survival.[3]

About 70% of patients with GISTs present with symptoms related to an enlarging abdominal mass, bleeding, or obstruction, with bleeding being the most common presenting symptom.[8–10] The incidental finding of a GIST at the time of endoscopy or surgery is also not uncommon, occurring in about 20% of patients.[9] At the time of presentation, as many as 50% of patients with GISTs present with distant metastases.[7] Of the patients who present with distant metastases, about two-thirds have

The authors have nothing to disclose.
Helen F. Graham Cancer Center, Department of Surgery, Christiana Care Health Services, 4701 Ogletown-Stanton Road, Suite 4000, Newark, DE 19713, USA
* Corresponding author.
E-mail address: jobennett@christianacare.org

Surg Oncol Clin N Am 21 (2012) 21–33
doi:10.1016/j.soc.2011.09.008
1055-3207/12/$ – see front matter © 2012 Elsevier Inc. All rights reserved.

hepatic involvement. Patients present with extra-abdominal metastases or lymph node involvement much less commonly, less than 10% of the time. In one series of 200 patients, 30% of patients who presented with metastatic disease were able to undergo complete resection.[7]

PREOPERATIVE IMAGING

Computed tomography (CT) scan is often the first imaging test used to evaluate a suspected intra-abdominal mass. CT can provide rapid and reproducible assessment of the size of the primary tumor and the relationship to surrounding structures.[11] CT scan is also a useful method for evaluating metastatic disease and for determining resectable versus unresectable tumors. Small tumors are usually well circumscribed and of low soft tissue density on unenhanced CT scans.[11] With intravenous contrast, these tumors typically show homogeneous enhancement. As the tumors get larger, they tend to show a patchy enhancement pattern with varying degrees of necrosis within the mass. CT scan can also identify the presence of metastatic lesions and is a useful tool for following lesions being treated with targeted therapy.

Magnetic resonance imaging (MRI) features of GIST are variable depending on the degree of necrosis and hemorrhage within the tumor.[12] These tumors typically enhance with intravenous gadolinium and have low signal intensity on T1 weighted images and high signal intensity on T2 weighted images. MRI is mainly indicated when liver metastases are suspected, specifically to assess resectability and to differentiate from other types of liver lesions.

Endoscopic ultrasound (EUS) biopsy has become the preferred method for obtaining a tissue diagnosis for tumors in the upper gastrointestinal tract that are accessible by endoscopy. Biopsy may not be necessary if the tumor has classic endoscopic findings and is easily resectable, but should be performed before initiating preoperative targeted therapy.[13] EUS and biopsy are also not indicated if the suspected GIST is symptomatic, as any bleeding or obstructing gastrointestinal tumor should be resected if the patient can tolerate surgery. The sensitivity of EUS fine-needle aspiration (FNA) cytology for GIST is dependent on tumor size, shape, and layer of origin.[14] EUS-FNA has a higher sensitivity for tumors in the stomach when compared with tumors of the duodenum.

STAGING

Staging of GISTs of the stomach is based on the tumor, node, metastases (TNM) staging system for sarcoma. The most important components of the staging of GISTs are tumor size and histologic grade. Stage I tumors are those smaller than 10 cm with a low mitotic rate (<5 mitoses/50 high-power field [hpf]). Stage II tumors include tumors smaller than 5 cm with high mitotic rate (>5 mitoses/50 hpf), as well as tumors larger than 10 cm with a low mitotic rate. Stage III tumors are those larger than 5 cm with a high mitotic rate, and stage IV tumors include those with lymphatic or distant metastases.[15] Although tumor size and mitotic rate are 2 of the most important prognostic features, other tumor characteristics have shown prognostic significance. Male sex, nongastric primary tumor location, R1/R2 resection, and epithelioid or mixed cell pathologic subtype have also been shown to be negative prognostic features.[16,17]

Miettinen and Lasota[18] developed a stratification for risk of progressive disease based on tumor size, mitotic index, and anatomic location. This risk stratification was based on long-term follow-up studies on 1,055 gastric, 629 small intestinal, 144 duodenal, and 111 rectal GISTs. For example, based on this risk stratification, a patient with a 6 cm gastric GIST with more than 5 mitosis/hpf would have a 16%

risk for progressive disease on long-term follow-up; however, a patient with a 6 cm jejunal GIST with more than 5 mitoses/hpf would have a 73% risk for progressive disease on long-term follow-up. This stratification system has been helpful in determining patient selection for adjuvant imatinib mesylate (STI-571; Gleevec) after curative resection.

PATHOLOGY

On gross examination, GISTs vary greatly in size and can become quite large, larger than 20 cm in diameter.[19] They often appear as a friable mass originating from the muscle rather than the epithelium of the GI tract. These tumors are often well circumscribed and unencapsulated; however, a pseudocapsule is occasionally present. Larger tumors may show cystic degeneration, necrosis, and focal hemorrhage.

Microscopically, most GISTs have a relatively uniform appearance, with most displaying a spindle cell type (70%).[5] The next most common type is the epithelioid type (20%), with the remainder of cases displaying either a mixed pattern or, less commonly, a ganglioma like or carcinoid like growth pattern. Tumors displaying a mixed cell type may show an abrupt transition between spindle cell and epithelioid areas, or may have more complex mixing of these cell types throughout the tumor.

The defining characteristic of GISTs is the presence of the cell-surface antigen CD117 receptor tyrosine kinase (KIT) identified by immunohistochemistry.[2] KIT is a growth factor transmembrane receptor that is the product of the proto-oncogene c-kit located on chromosome 4.[19] KIT is activated by its ligand stem-cell factor, leading to proliferation, adhesion, apoptosis, and differentiation.[2] KIT is closely related to other receptors in the family of tyrosine kinase receptors (TKRs), including platelet-derived growth factor receptor (PDGFR).[19] CD34 is a hematopoietic progenitor cell antigen that is positive in 70% to 80% of GISTs. It is more commonly positive in GISTs of the esophagus and rectum compared with the stomach and small intestine.[19]

MOLECULAR ANALYSIS

KIT mutations are common in GISTs, occurring about 90% to 95% of the time.[19,20] KIT is a transmembrane tyrosine kinase receptor present in many germ cells, hematopoietic stem cells, and in the interstitial cells of Cajal (ICC). Its ligand is stem cell factor, also known as the Kit ligand. Activation of KIT leads to many complex downstream cascades that regulate cell function, proliferation, differentiation, and control of apoptosis.[21] KIT mutation results in constitutive activation of multiple kinase pathways and is believed to be among the earliest changes that promote malignant transformation of ICC to GIST.[22] KIT is in the same tyrosine kinase receptor family as PDGFR alpha (PDGFRA), and when KIT mutations are not present, PDGFRA mutations have been discovered (5% of GISTs).[23]

The most common KIT mutation occurs in exon 11 (50%–70%).[19] Exon 11 mutations occur more commonly among low-risk patients. Patients with exon 11 mutations typically show a longer event-free and overall survival. They also have a higher response to targeted therapy and a longer time to progression than those with other mutations.[19] Exon 9 mutations occur in 10% to 18% of GISTs and are seen more frequently in higher-risk GISTs. GISTs with exon 9 mutations are biologically more aggressive then GISTs with other mutations.[24] A small subset of GISTs (~10%) displays a wild-type KIT with no identifiable mutation.[19,20] About one-third of these tumors will harbor mutations in the PDGFRA gene.[25] PDGFRA mutations show a strong predilection to gastric GIST with epithelioid morphology.[26] These mutations can explain the response to targeted therapy seen in patients lacking KIT mutations, as is discussed later.[20]

TECHNIQUES OF LAPAROSCOPIC AND OPEN RESECTION

Surgical resection remains the treatment of choice for GISTs.[27] Historically, surgical resection involved a goal of achieving 1-cm to 2-cm negative margins to minimize the risk of local recurrence.[28,29] DeMatteo and colleagues[7] recently showed in a prospective review of 200 patients that tumor size, but not microscopic margins of resection, predicted survival. The goal for surgical resection is now widely accepted to be negative gross margins.[7,27] This study also showed that GISTs rarely metastasize to locoregional lymph nodes and, unlike gastric adenocarcinoma, lymph node dissection in the treatment of gastric GISTs is not necessary.

The realization that wide surgical margins and extensive lymphadenectomies were not indicated increased interest in laparoscopic resection. The safety of minimally invasive techniques for the resection of gastric GISTs has been proven in several series. Novitsky and colleagues[28] reported a series of 50 patients who underwent laparoscopic or laparoendoscopic resection of gastric GISTs. They were able to achieve negative margins in all cases with no local or port-site recurrences at 36 months of follow-up. A similar series of 51 patients with gastric GIST treated by laparoscopic resection was reported by Choi and colleagues.[30] They reported no reoperation or operative mortality and found no local recurrences at 60 months of follow-up. There was 1 postoperative complication encountered in a patient with delayed gastric emptying but no major postoperative complications, such as bleeding, leaks, obstruction, or abscess formation.

In a comparison of laparoscopic to open resection for gastric GIST, Matthews and colleagues[29] found no difference in operative time, estimated blood loss, or tumor size, but did note a significant difference in length of stay in the laparoscopic group (3.8 days) compared with the open group (6.2 days). They found no trocar site recurrences and concluded that the laparoscopic approach was safe and appropriate. In this series, laparoscopic resections included wedge resections, partial gastrectomies, and transgastric needlescopic enucleations.

Matthews and colleagues[29] described several techniques for laparoscopic wedge resection of gastric GIST in this series, depending on the tumor size and location. Tumor position was confirmed by transillumination with intraoperative esophagogastroduodenoscopy (EGD) and bimanual palpation with graspers. Laparoscopic ultrasound was also used to confirm tumor position and to survey the liver for metastatic disease. Small tumors were then excised with a gastrointestinal anastomosis (GIA) stapler. Larger tumors were resected using ultrasonic coagulating shears and the gastrotomy was then closed with either intracorporeal suturing or with a GIA stapler. For large tumors, or tumors near the pylorus, where wedge resection would result in narrowing of the gastric lumen, a partial gastrectomy was performed. All tumors were removed in an endoscopic retrieval bag.

Several techniques have been described for laparoscopic resection of gastric GIST of the posterior wall of the stomach. One method involves approaching the lesion through the anterior wall of the stomach.[28,29] In this approach, a gastrotomy is made with ultrasonic coagulating shears on the anterior gastric wall after the tumor is located with intraoperative EGD. The lesion of the posterior wall is then elevated using partial-thickness stay sutures and resected with an endoscopic GIA stapler. Finally, the anterior gastrotomy is closed with an endoscopic GIA stapler. Another technique for resection of gastric GISTs of the posterior gastric wall is to approach the lesion through the lesser sac by dividing the gastrocolic omentum and short gastric vessels.[28] The lesion can then be resected in a manner similar to anterior wall lesions.

Matthews and colleagues[29] also described a percutaneous, transgastric needle-scopic approach of resecting GISTs of the gastroesophageal junction. In this technique, the abdominal cavity is first insufflated using a 2-mm needlescopic umbilical port. Two additional 2-mm ports are placed and inserted through the gastric wall under combined needlescopic and endoscopic guidance. The abdomen is then desufflated and the remainder of the procedure is performed under endoscopic guidance. Epinephrine is then injected into the submucosa circumferentially around the tumor. The mucosa is incised and the tumor is enucleated from the underlying muscularis using an endoloop. The tumor is then removed through the mouth using an endoscopic snare.

ADJUVANT TARGETED THERAPY

GISTs metastasize primarily to the peritoneal cavity and/or the liver. Lymphatic metas-tases are rare and usually represent end-stage disease. Conventional chemotherapy and radiation therapy has historically been of little value in treating GISTs.[31] Previ-ously, surgical resection of recurrent or metastatic disease was the only treatment option, but the results were poor with nearly all patients developing recurrent disease with short disease-free intervals.[27,32]

Imatinib mesylate (STI-571; Gleevec) is a 2-phenlypyrimidine derivative that inhibits the binding of adenosine triphosphate (ATP) to ABL kinase.[27] Imatinib was initially developed to treat leukemia by blocking the BCR-ABL oncogene. Imatinib, however, is not specific for ABL and has significant inhibitory activity against both KIT and PDGFRA. In 2000, imatinib was therefore used as compassionate therapy in a patient with advanced metastatic GIST.[33] This patient had a complete metabolic response, with no residual activity on positron emission tomography scan and 50% reduced tumor volume on MRI, after 1 month of therapy. The success of this patient sparked further interest in investigating the use of imatinib as a treatment for GISTs in phase I/II clinical trials.

The American College of Surgeons Oncology Group (ACOSOG) conducted a phase II trial to evaluate the benefit of imatinib in the adjuvant setting (400 mg/d for 1 year) in high-risk patients (tumor ≥10 cm in size, tumor rupture, <5 peritoneal metastases) who have undergone complete resection of a KIT expressing primary GIST (ACOSOG Z9000).[34] Before the availability of imatinib, patients with high-risk primary GISTs were reported to have a 2-year survival of approximately 50%.[34] There were 107 patients enrolled in the study and at a median follow-up of 4 years, and the 1-year, 2-year, and 3-year survival rates were 99%, 97%, and 97%. The 1-year, 2-year, and 3-year recurrence-free survival rates were 94%, 73%, and 61%.

A randomized phase III study (ACOSOG Z9001) compared the use of adjuvant ima-tinib (400 mg/d for 1 year) to placebo for patients with moderate-risk tumors (≥3 cm) who underwent complete resection.[35] Accrual was stopped early in this trial because of a statistically significant improvement in recurrence-free survival in the imatinib group. Recurrence-free survival at 1 year in the imatinib arm was 97% compared with 83% in the placebo arm. There was no difference in overall survival in the short-term follow-up data, but these patients will continue to be followed for 10 years and long-term follow-up data are not yet available. Importantly, the investigators also showed that the rate of recurrence seemed to increase approximately 18 months after surgery, or 6 months after completion of the study therapy. The recurrence-free survival curves between imatinib-treated patients and the placebo group diverge so long as patients are receiving imatinib, but shortly after drug cessation (1 year) the curves converge and any benefit from imatinib is then lost. These results are consistent with a trial in metastatic GIST by Blay and colleagues,[36] which showed that patients with responding or stable disease on imatinib developed tumor progression after a median of 6 months after randomization to discontinuation of therapy. The benefit of imatinib does not seem to be durable after patients are taken off therapy and when given for 1 year or less. This raised significant interest in evaluating longer-term adjuvant therapy to further prolong recurrence-free survival and to determine if any overall survival benefit can be achieved.

The Scandinavian Sarcoma Group (SSG) and the Sarcoma Group of the Arbeitsgemeinschaft Internistische Onkologie (AIO) conducted a prospective multicenter phase III trial comparing adjuvant imatinib therapy for 3 years versus 1 year.[37] This trial included 400 patients who were considered to be at high risk for recurrence despite complete resection with a median follow-up of 54 months. High-risk patients were defined as those with tumors larger than 10 cm, more than 10 mitoses per 50 hpf, tumors that were both larger than 5 cm with more than 5 mitoses per 50 hpf, or intraoperative tumor spillage. The results showed that at 5 years, 66% of patients taking imatinib for 3 years remained free of cancer compared with 48% who had received adjuvant imatinib for only 1 year (P<.0001). Importantly, this is the first prospective phase III trial demonstrating an overall survival benefit from imatinib in the adjuvant setting. In this trial, overall survival was 92% for patients taking imatinib for 3 years compared with 82% who received imatinib for only 1 year (P = .019).

The efficacy of using imatinib at higher dosing levels has also been investigated. Verweij and colleagues[38] randomly assigned 946 patients to receive imatinib 400 mg either once or twice per day. They showed that there was no difference between the 2 groups in complete or partial response. There was, however, a significant difference between the 2 groups in progression-free survival, 50% versus 56% (P = .026), when comparing once to twice per day. Another randomized trial, by Demetri and colleagues,[39] assigned patients to receive imatinib 400 mg per day or 600 mg per day. They found no difference between the 2 groups in any of the efficacy end points.

The role for high-dose imatinib was addressed in a multicenter phase III randomized trial in 2008.[40] In this trial, 748 patients with advanced unresectable or metastatic GISTs from 148 centers in the United States and Canada were randomized to receive imatinib 400 mg once or twice per day. There were no significant differences between the 2 groups in response rates, progression-free survival, or overall survival. The study also showed that 33% of patients who had disease progression on standard dose imatinib and crossed over to the high-dose group achieved either an objective response or stable disease. The investigators concluded, based on these results, that imatinib therapy should be initiated at 400 mg per day with a consideration for dose escalation on progression of disease.

The indications for the use of imatinib as adjuvant therapy based on these trials include patients with positive margins, unresectable metastatic disease, and those with high-risk tumors. Although it has been shown that both size and mitotic figures (>5 mitoses/50 hpf) are important prognostic features, the exact size criteria for using adjuvant imatinib has not been clearly defined. According to the National Comprehensive Cancer Network Guidelines, a tumor with both size larger than 5 cm and more than 5 mitoses per 50 hpf is high risk and meets criteria for using adjuvant imatinib.[13] In the ACOSOG Z9000 trial, high-risk tumors were defined as tumors 10 cm or larger in size,[34] and in the ACOSOG Z9001 trial, there was a benefit in recurrence-free survival with adjuvant imatinib in moderate-risk tumors of 3 cm or larger.[35] The SSG/AOI trial defined high-risk tumors as those larger than 10 cm, more than 10 mitoses per 50 hpf, or tumors both 5 cm or larger and 5 or more mitoses per 50 hpf.[37] For patients who have borderline-risk tumors based on the variable definitions for high-risk tumors, individual clinical discretion must be used to determine the appropriateness of adjuvant therapy.

NEOADJUVANT TARGETED THERAPY

Imatinib is also being investigated in the neoadjuvant setting. Raut and colleagues[41] conducted a retrospective analysis of 69 patients with locally advanced primary or metastatic GIST treated with neoadjuvant imatinib. They found that response to therapy strongly correlated with surgical outcome. Complete surgical resection was achieved in only 25% of patients who demonstrated limited disease progression after neoadjuvant therapy, and in only 7% of patients who showed full disease progression. These results indicated that there seems to be a role for imatinib followed by surgery in the 68% of patients who had stable disease on neoadjuvant therapy; however, the role of imatinib followed by surgery in patients who had disease progression on neoadjuvant therapy seems to be limited. The 12-month progression-free and overall survival were poor for patients who had full progression on imatinib, both 0%, whereas responders demonstrated 80% progression-free survival and 95% overall survival during the same 12 months.

Andtbacka and colleagues[42] investigated the use of imatinib before surgery in a high-risk group of patients with locally advanced primary, recurrent, or metastatic GIST. The duration of neoadjuvant therapy was determined based on the radiographic response. Patients underwent surgical resection after there was no change in tumor size or enhancement on 2 consecutive radiographic studies 2 to 3 months apart. In patients who showed evidence of tumor progression, the dose of imatinib was initially increased, and if there was evidence of continued progression, they underwent surgical resection. Of the 47 patients in this study, 11 patients were treated for locally advanced GIST and all were able to undergo complete resection; however, 35 patients were treated for recurrent or metastatic GIST and only 11 were able to undergo complete resection. Patients who had even a partial response to therapy were more likely to undergo complete surgical resection, which in turn led to improved survival.

The Radiation Therapy Oncology Group S0132 trial is a prospective phase II trial evaluating the use of imatinib in primary GIST or as a preoperative cytoreduction agent for metastatic GIST.[43] Early results from this trial showed a 2-year progression-free survival of 83% in patients with advanced primary GIST ($\geq$5 cm) and 77% in patients with metastatic or recurrent GIST ($\geq$2 cm). Overall survival was 93% in patients with advanced primary GIST and 91% in patients with metastatic or recurrent GIST. Importantly, there was no increased rate of surgical complications noted in this population of patients receiving neoadjuvant imatinib. Follow-up results of this trial are pending.

Although it seems logical to use imatinib in the neoadjuvant setting for locally advanced unresectable tumors, one difficulty in interpreting the data for this group of patients is the lack of a clear definition of an unresectable tumor. Without a clear definition, patients who may be considered unresectable by one institution might be considered resectable at another institution. For patients who will need multiorgan resection, especially when morbidity may be high, it is reasonable to use imatinib preoperatively as a means to select patients who will be responders and who will likely demonstrate improved survival. For patients with metastatic disease, imatinib can also be used after resection of the primary tumor and before metastasectomy. The true role for targeted therapy followed by surgery for patients with metastatic GIST needs to be further investigated in the setting of randomized trials.

RESISTANCE TO TARGETED THERAPY

Imatinib resistance has become a significant concern in the treatment of GISTs. As many as 9% to 13% of patients will have an initial resistance to imatinib and patients who respond to imatinib may develop an acquired resistance.[38,39,44,45] Secondary resistance develops in most patients at a median of 2 years of therapy.[46] The exact mechanism for the development of resistance to imatinib is unclear but there are several possibilities. There is evidence that the oral bioavailability of imatinib decreases in patients with chronic use.[44] Resistance may also develop through secondary KIT mutations[47] or by activating genes that control the downstream signal transduction pathways of KIT.[44]

Other kinase inhibitors are being investigated to treat patients with resistance to imatinib (Table 1). Sunitinib is a small-molecule tyrosine kinase inhibitor (TKI) with inhibitory activity against c-KIT and vascular endothelial growth factor receptors (VEGFRs).[48] Sunitinib has been shown to have activity against imatinib-resistant GISTs. Results of a phase I/II continuation trial presented in 2005 for patients with imatinib-resistant disease evaluated 97 patients on several dose regimens of sunitinib.[49] Partial response by RECIST (Response Evaluation Criteria In Solid Tumor) criteria or stable disease for a period of more than 6 months was seen in 32 patients who were entered into the continuation study. With 2 to 3 years of data, median time to progression was 8 months with an overall median survival of 20 months. As with imatinib therapy, KIT mutation status seems to be important in predicting a response to sunitinib. Unlike imatinib, however, patients with wild-type KIT or exon 9 mutations seem to have longer median time to progression than patients with exon 11 mutations. Median overall survival was also shorter in patients with exon 11 mutations.

There has been one completed phase III double-blind randomized trial comparing sunitinib to placebo in patients with imatinib intolerance or resistant disease.[50] This was a multicenter European study that showed a significant difference in median

Table 1
Tyrosine kinase inhibitors for the treatment of GIST

Drug	Target	Current Phase of Investigationd
Imatinib mesylate (Gleevec)	KIT, PDGFRA, BCR-ABL[27,52]	Phase III[35,37] Approved for use in GIST[52]
Sunitinib (Sutent)	KIT, VEGFR, PDGFR, RET, FLT-3[48,52]	Phase III[50,51] Approved for use in GIST[52]
Nilotinib (Tasigna)	BCR-ABL, KIT, PDGFR[52]	Phase III[52]
Masitinib	KIT, PDGFR, LYN[52]	Phase III[52]
Dasatinib (Sprycel)	KIT, BCR-ABL, SRC, BTK, FAK[52]	Phase II[52]
Sorafenib (Nexavar)	KIT, VEGFR, PDGFR, BRAF, FLT-3, Raf-1[52]	Phase II[52]

Abbreviations: BCR-ABL, oncogene fusion protein; BRAF, serine/threonine protein kinase; FAK, focal adhesion kinase; FLT-3, Fms-like tyrosine kinase 3; GIST, gastrointestinal stromal tumor; KIT, cell-surface antigen CD117 receptor tyrosine kinase; LYN, member of the src family of tyrosine kinases; PDGFR, platelet-derived growth factor receptor; Raf-1, proto-oncogene serine/threonine protein kinase. RET, proto-oncogene, encodes receptor tyrosine kinase; SRC, proto-oncogene tyrosine protein kinase; VEGFR, vascular endothelial growth factor receptor, time to progression in patients treated with sunitinib (6 months) compared with placebo (1.5 months). Partial tumor response was seen in 8% of patients in the sunitinib group compared with 0% in the placebo group. Updated results from this study were published in 2006 and showed a continuation of the initial trends with a significantly greater overall survival ($P = .007$) in the treatment arm with a higher proportion of stable disease or partial response compared with the placebo arm.[51]

Although imatinib and sunitinib are the only 2 agents that have been approved for the treatment of GISTs, several other agents are currently under investigation (see **Table 1**). Nilotinib is a BCR-ABL kinase inhibitor with more potency than imatinib.[52] Results of a phase I study of nilotinib in combination with imatinib in a subset of patients with advanced GIST resistant to imatinib and sunitinib showed evidence of clinical benefit with a median progression-free survival of 12 weeks and median overall survival of 34 weeks.[46,53] Nilotinib is now being investigated in phase III trials both as initial therapy in comparison with imatinib and as treatment for disease that is resistant to both imatinib and sunitinib in comparison with best supportive care.[52] Masitinib is a TKI with greater activity than imatinib against the wild-type KIT receptor. In a phase II study of imatinib-naïve patients with locally advanced or metastatic GIST, treatment with masitinib resulted in a complete response in 1 of 30 patients, a partial response in 15 of 30 patients, stable disease in 13 of 30 patients, and progression of disease in 1 of 30 patients.[54] These results have led to the initiation of a phase III trial comparing imatinib to masitinib as first-line therapy in patients with unresectable locally advanced, metastatic, or recurrent GIST. Dasatinib (Sprycel) is a multikinase inhibitor with activity against SRC, SRC-related kinases, and the tyrosine kinases BTK and FAK.[52] At higher concentrations, it also has activity against BCR-ABL and KIT. Dasatinib is currently being investigated in a phase II study as first-line therapy in patients with GIST.[55] Sorafenib (Nexavar) is a multikinase inhibitor with activity against KIT, VEGFR, PDGFR, and serine/threonine kinases.[52] The use of sorafenib as a fourth-line agent in patients who failed to be controlled by imatinib, sunitinib, and nilotinib was recently evaluated in retrospective analysis of 32 patients and showed promising results. Further investigation into the use of sorafenib in the management of GISTs is under way.

SUMMARY

Gastrointestinal stromal tumors are relatively rare tumors, with between 5,000[4] and 10,000[5] new cases per year in the United States. The most common primary site is the stomach (50%), followed by the small intestine (36%), colon (7%), rectum (5%), and esophagus (1%).[3] KIT mutations are common in GISTs, occurring about 90% of the time.[19,20] The most common mutation occurs in exon 11 (50%–70%),[19] and these mutations occur more commonly among low-risk patients. Exon 9 mutations occur in 10% to 18% of GISTs and are seen more frequently in higher-risk GISTs. The only current option for cure is complete surgical resection. Studies have shown that complete resection of all gross disease without need for radical margins and without lymphadenectomy is optimal therapy. This has led to interest in laparoscopic resection. The safety of minimally invasive techniques for the resection of gastric GISTs has been proven in several series.

Imatinib is a small-molecule tyrosine kinase inhibitor with inhibitory activity against both KIT and PDGFRA.[27] Imatinib was shown to improve progression-free survival in the adjuvant setting after 1 year of therapy; however, a recent prospective multicenter phase III trial has shown that 3 years of imatinib therapy (vs 1 year) improves overall survival as well.[37] In this trial, overall survival was 92% for patients taking imatinib for 3 years compared with 82% for patients who received imatinib for only 1 year

($P = .019$). Imatinib is also being investigated in the neoadjuvant setting to downstage unresectable tumors to resectable, as selection criteria to choose patients who will respond to therapy and, hence, benefit from extensive surgery, and as a bridge after resecting the primary tumor and before metastasectomy. The role for using imatinib in the neoadjuvant setting has not been clearly defined and such cases should be handled by a multidisciplinary team with surgeons and medical oncologists with expertise in treating GISTs.

Imatinib resistance has become a significant concern in the treatment of GIST. As many as 9% to 13% of patients will have an initial resistance to imatinib, and patients who respond to imatinib may develop an acquired resistance.[38,39,44,45] Secondary resistance develops in most patients at a median of 2 years of therapy.[43] Other small-molecule kinase inhibitors are under investigation and upcoming clinical trials will hopefully give patients more options for improved outcome.

REFERENCES

1. Kindblom LG, Remotti HE, Aldenborg F, et al. Gastrointestinal pacemaker cell tumor (GIPACT): gastrointestinal stromal tumors show phenotypic characteristics of the interstitial cells of Cajal. Am J Pathol 1998;152(5):1259–69.
2. Hirota S, Isozaki K, Moriyama Y, et al. Gain-or-function mutations of c-kit in human gastrointestinal stromal tumors. Science 1998;279:577–80.
3. Tran T, Davila JA, El-Serag HB. The epidemiology of malignant gastrointestinal stromal tumors: an analysis of 1,458 cases from 1992 to 2000. Am J Gastroenterol 2005;100(1):162–8.
4. Blanke CD, Eisenberg BL, Heinrich MC. Gastrointestinal stromal tumors. Curr Treat Options Oncol 2001;2(6):485–91.
5. Fletcher CDM, Berman JJ, Corless C, et al. Diagnosis of gastrointestinal stromal tumors: a consensus approach. Hum Pathol 2002;33(5):459–65.
6. Emory TS, Sobin LH, Lukes L, et al. Prognosis of gastrointestinal smooth-muscle (stromal) tumors: dependence on anatomic site. Am J Surg Pathol 1999;23(1):82–7.
7. DeMatteo RP, Lewis JJ, Leung D, et al. Two hundred gastrointestinal stromal tumors. Ann Surg 2000;231(1):51–8.
8. Roberts PJ, Eisenberg B. Clinical presentation of gastrointestinal stromal tumors and treatment of operable disease. Eur J Cancer 2002;38(S5):S37–8.
9. Nilsson B, Bumming P, Meis-Kindblom JM, et al. Gatrointestinal stromal tumors: the incidence, prevalence, clinical course, and prognostication in the pre imatinib mesylate era. Cancer 2005;103(4):821–9.
10. Hueman MT, Schulick RD. Management of gastrointestinal stromal tumors. Surg Clin North Am 2008;88:599–614.
11. King MD. The radiology of gastrointestinal stromal tumors (GIST). Cancer Imaging 2005;5:150–6.
12. Levy AD, Remotti HE, Thompson WM, et al. Gastrointestinal stromal tumors: radiologic features with pathologic correlation. Radiographics 2003;23(2):283–304, 456 [quiz: 532].
13. Von Mehren M, Benjamin RS, Bui MM. NCCN clinical practice guidelines in oncology (NCCN Guidelines): soft tissue sarcoma. Version 1.2011:MS15–MS23. 2011. Available at: http://www.nccn.org/professionals/physician_gls/pdf/sarcoma.pdf. Accessed April 23, 2011.

14. Sepe PS, Moparty B, Pitman MB, et al. EUS-guided FNA for the diagnosis of GI stromal cell tumors: sensitivity and cytologic yield. Gastrointest Endosc 2009; 70(2):254–61.
15. Edge SB, Byrd DR, Compton CC, et al, editors. AJCC cancer staging manual. 7th edition. New York (NY): Springer; 2010. p. 175–80.
16. Rutkowski P, Nowecki ZI, Michej W, et al. Risk criteria and prognostic factors for predicting recurrences after resection of primary gastrointestinal stromal tumor. Ann Surg Oncol 2007;14(7):2018–27.
17. Fujimoto Y, Nakanishi Y, Yoshimura K, et al. Clinicopathologic study of primary malignant gastrointestinal stromal tumor of the stomach, with special reference to prognostic factors: analysis of results in 140 surgically resected patients. Gastric Cancer 2003;6:39–48.
18. Miettinen M, Lasota J. Gastrointestinal stromal tumors: pathology and prognosis at different sites. Semin Diagn Pathol 2006;23(2):70–83.
19. Badalamenti G, Rodolico V, Fulfaro F, et al. Gastrointestinal stromal tumors (GISTs): focus on histopathological diagnosis and biomolecular features. Ann Oncol 2007;18:vi136–40.
20. Heinrich MC, Corless CL, Demetri GD, et al. Kinase mutations and imatinib response in patients with metastatic gastrointestinal stromal tumor. J Clin Oncol 2003;21(23):4342–9.
21. D'Amato G, Steinert DM, McAuliffe JC, et al. Update on the biology and therapy of gastrointestinal stromal tumors. Cancer Control 2005;12(1):44–56.
22. Taylor ML, Metcalfe DD. Kit signal transduction. Hematol Oncol Clin North Am 2000;14(3):517–35.
23. Qiu FH, Ray P, Barker PE, et al. Primary structure of c-kit: relationship with the CSF-1/PDGF receptor kinase family—oncogenic activation of v-kit involves deletion of extracellular domain and C terminus. EMBO J 1998;7(4):1003–11.
24. Corless CL, Fletcher JA, Heinrich MC. Biology of gastrointestinal stromal tumors. J Clin Oncol 2004;22(18):3813–25.
25. Rubin BP, Heinrich MC, Corless CL. Gastrointestinal stromal tumour. Lancet 2007; 369(9574):1731–41.
26. Miettinen M, Lasota J. Gastrointestinal stromal tumors: review on morphology, molecular pathology, prognosis, and differential diagnosis. Arch Pathol Lab Med 2006;130:1466–78.
27. Heinrich MC, Corless CL. Gastric GI stromal tumors (GISTs): the role of surgery in the era of targeted therapy. J Surg Oncol 2005;90(3):195–207.
28. Novitsky YW, Kercher KW, Sing RF, et al. Long-term outcomes of laparoscopic resection of gastric gastrointestinal stromal tumors. Ann Surg 2006;243(6): 738–47.
29. Matthews BD, Walsh RM, Kercher KW, et al. Laparoscopic vs open resection of gastric stromal tumors. Surg Endosc 2002;16(5):803–7.
30. Choi SM, Kim MC, Jung GJ, et al. Laparoscopic wedge resection for gastric GIST: long-term follow-up results. Eur J Surg Oncol 2007;33(4):444–7.
31. DeMatteo RP, Heinrich MC, El-Rifai WM, et al. Clinical management of gastrointestinal stromal tumors: before and after STI-571. Hum Pathol 2002;33(5): 466–77.
32. Ng EH, Pollock RE, Romsdahl MM. Prognostic implications of patterns of failure for gastrointestinal leiomyosarcomas. Cancer 1992;69:1334–41.
33. Joensuu H, Roberts PJ, Sarlomo-Rikala M, et al. Effect of the tyrosine kinase inhibitor STI571 in a patient with metastatic gastrointestinal stromal tumor. N Engl J Med 2001;344(14):1052–6.

34. DeMatteo RP, Owzar K, Antonescu CR, et al. Efficacy of adjuvant imatinib mesylate following complete resection of localized, primary gastrointestinal stromal tumor (GIST) at high risk of recurrence: the US intergroup phase II trial ACOSOG Z9000 (abstract). Data presented at the 2008 ASCO Gastrointestinal Cancers Symposium. Orlando (FL), January 25–27, 2008.
35. DeMatteo RP, Ballman KV, Antonescu CR, et al. Placebo-controlled randomized trial of adjuvant imatinib mesylate following the resection of localized, primary gastrointestinal stromal tumor (GIST). Lancet 2009;373:1097–104.
36. Blay JY, Le Cesne A, Ray-Coquard I, et al. Prospective multicentric randomized phase III study of imatinib in patients with advanced gastrointestinal stromal tumors comparing interruption versus continuation of treatment beyond 1 year: the French Sarcoma Group. J Clin Oncol 2007;25(9):1107–13.
37. Joensuu H, Erikson M, Hatrmann J, et al. Twelve vs 36 months of adjuvant imatinib (IM) as treatment of operable GIST with a high risk of recurrence: final results of a randomized trial (SSGXVIII/AIO). 47th Annual Meeting of the American Society of Clinical Oncology. Abstract No. LBA1. Chicago (IL): June 5, 2011.
38. Verweij J, Casali PG, Zalcberg J, et al. Progression-free survival in gastrointestinal stromal tumours with high-dose imatinib: randomised trial. Lancet 2004; 364(9440):1127–34.
39. Demetri GD, von Mehren M, Blanke CD, et al. Efficacy and safety of imatinib mesylate in advanced gastrointestinal stromal tumors. N Engl J Med 2002;347(7): 472–80.
40. Blanke CD, Rankin C, Demetri GD. Phase III randomized, intergroup trial assessing imatinib mesylate at two dose levels in patients with unresectable or metastatic gastrointestinal stromal tumors expressing the KIT receptor tyrosine kinase: S0033. J Clin Oncol 2008;26(4):626–32.
41. Raut CP, Posner M, Desai J, et al. Surgical management of advanced gastrointestinal stromal tumors after treatment with targeted systemic therapy using kinase inhibitors. J Clin Oncol 2006;24(15):2325–31.
42. Andtbacka RH, Ng CS, Scaife CL, et al. Surgical resection of gastrointestinal stromal tumors after treatment with imatinib. Ann Surg Oncol 2007;14(1): 14–24.
43. Eisenberg BL, Harris J, Blanke CD, et al. Phase II trial of neoadjuvant/adjuvant imatinib mesylate (IM) for advanced primary and metastatic/recurrent operable gastrointestinal stromal tumor (GIST): early results of RTOG 0132/ACIN 6665. J Surg Oncol 2009;99:42–7.
44. Bickenbach K, Wilcox R, Veerapong J, et al. A review of resistance patterns and phenotypic changes in gastrointestinal stromal tumors following imatinib mesylate therapy. J Gastrointest Surg 2007;11(6):758–66.
45. Van Oosterom AT, Judson I, Verweij J, et al. Safety and efficacy of imatinib (STI571) in metastatic gastrointestinal stromal tumours: a phase I study. Lancet 2001;358(9291):1421–3.
46. Demetri GD, Casali PG, Blay JY, et al. A phase I study of single-agent nilotinib or in combination with imatinib in patients with imatinib-resistant gastrointestinal stromal tumors. Clin Cancer Res 2009;15(18):5910–6.
47. Antonescu CR, Besmer P, Guo T, et al. Acquired resistance to imatinib in gastrointestinal stromal tumor occurs through secondary gene mutation. Clin Cancer Res 2005;11:4182–90.
48. Hopkins TG, Marples M, Stark D. Sunitinib in the management of gastrointestinal stromal tumors (GISTs). Eur J Surg Oncol 2008;34(8):844–50.

49. Maki R, Fletcher J, Heinrich M, et al. Results from a continuation trial of SU11248 in patients with imatinib resistant gastrointestinal stromal tumor (GIST). ASCO Annual Meeting Proceedings. J Clin Oncol 2005;23(16S):9011.

50. Therasse P, Arbuck SG, Eisenhauer EA, et al. New guidelines to evaluate the response to treatment in solid tumors. J Natl Cancer Inst 2000;92:205–16.

51. Demetri GD, van Oosterom AT, Garrett CR, et al. Efficacy and safety of sunitinib in patients with advanced gastrointestinal stromal tumour after failure of imatinib: a randomised controlled trial. Lancet 2006;368:1329–38.

52. Demetri GD. Differential properties of current tyrosine kinase inhibitors in gastrointestinal stromal tumors. Semin Oncol 2011;38(2):S10–9.

53. Montemurro M, Schoffski P, Reichardt P, et al. Nilotinib in the treatment of advanced gastrointestinal stromal tumours resistant to both imatinib and sunitinib. Eur J Cancer 2009;45(13):2293–7.

54. Le Cesne A, Blay JY, Bui BN, et al. Phase II study of oral masitinib mesilate in imatinib-naïve patients with locally advanced or metastatic gastro-intestinal stromal tumour (GIST). Eur J Cancer 2010;46(8):1344–51.

55. Demetri GD, Lo RP, MacPherson IR, et al. Phase I dose-escalation and pharmacokinetic study of dasatinib in patients with advanced solid tumors. Clin Cancer Res 2009;15:6232–40.

Familial Gastric Cancer: Genetics, Diagnosis, and Management

Vanessa R. Blair, FRACS, PhD[a,b,*]

KEYWORDS

- Familial gastric cancer • Hereditary diffuse gastric cancer
- E-cadherin • Prophylactic gastrectomy

An army marches on its stomach.
      —*Napoleon Bonaparte 1769–1821*

The Bonapartes are probably the most notorious reported gastric cancer family. However, recent analysis of Napoleon's family history and pathology records challenges the assumption of inherited predisposition.[1] Two hundred years ago, the practice of medicine largely rested on the arts of taking an accurate history and sharp clinical observation. Today, despite the explosion in molecular and genetic knowledge, this is still the case and a meticulous family history remains a cornerstone of diagnosis in familial cancer.

Although hereditary diffuse gastric cancer (HDGC) is relatively rare, sporadic, gastric cancer, it is the fourth most common cancer worldwide. In 1998, germline mutations in the E-cadherin gene (*CDH1*) were first described in three gastric cancer families from New Zealand.[2] In the year after this discovery, different *CDH1* mutations were identified in other gastric cancer families from around the world, culminating in the definition of the first and, to date, only inherited cancer syndrome dominated by gastric cancer, HDGC.[3] Despite extensive mutation searching in other candidate genes, no further mutations have been found in families in which gastric cancer predominates.

Parry Guilford and colleagues[2] identified the mutant *CDH1* gene, in part, because the pedigree of the index family (a large Maori family known as Family A) was well

The author has nothing to disclose.
[a] Department of Surgery, Faculty of Medicine and Health Sciences, The University of Auckland, Private Bag 92019, Auckland 1142, New Zealand
[b] Department of Surgery, Whangarei Base Hospital, Hospital Road, Private Bag 9742, Whangarei 0148, New Zealand
* Corresponding author. Department of Surgery, Whangarei Base Hospital, Hospital Road, Private Bag 9742, Whangarei 0148, New Zealand.
E-mail address: vanessa.blair@northlanddhb.org.nz

documented, permitting an accurate genetic linkage analysis. Forty years before this, in 1964, Dr Ted Jones, a young resident doctor at Tauranga Hospital had published the tragic story of multiple deaths in very young family members from a diffuse type of stomach cancer.[4] In 1965, Pekka Lauren,[5] of the eponymous Lauren Classification, published his seminal work on the different morphologic types of gastric cancer.

Lauren described the distinction between stomach cancers that form glands (eg, cancers of the colonic intestine), which he called the "intestinal type," and the "diffuse type" in which discohesive malignant cells invade in single files, sheets, or nests of cells without forming a discrete mass. Epithelial-cadherin is a cell-to-cell adhesion molecule that is a central component of the adherens junction. The difference in E-cadherin expression between gastric cancer histotypes was first demonstrated immunohistochemically by Shimoyama and Hirohashi[6] in 1991. Their study showed that in diffuse gastric cancer (DGC) E-cadherin expression was occasionally absent, but more often reduced or abnormal. Subsequently, Becker and colleagues[7] supported this by demonstrating that CDH1 mutations are restricted to sporadic gastric cancers with diffuse morphology.

Later work demonstrated that inactivating E-cadherin mutations are exclusively observed in the diffuse component of mixed gastric carcinomas.[8] In a commentary on this paper and other literature, Chan and Wong[9] highlighted that loss of E-cadherin provides a "plausible explanation" for the divergent morphologic phenotype in lobular versus ductal breast cancer and DGC versus intestinal gastric cancer (IGC). In Newfoundland, Canada, a germline CDH1 mutation was detected in another very large family; however, they were originally identified as a breast cancer family.[10]

This article focuses on the diagnosis and management of familial gastric cancer, particularly HDGC. First, existing consensus guidelines are discussed and then the pathology and genetics of HDGC are reviewed. Second, patient management is covered, including surveillance gastroscopy, prophylactic total gastrectomy, and management of the risk of breast cancer.

CONSENSUS GUIDELINES

In 1999, the first guidelines on diagnosis and management of familial gastric cancer were published by the International Gastric Cancer Linkage Consortium (IGCLC).[11] In New Zealand, because of the particularly young age at which HDGC patients have died, guidelines were needed on the youngest age at which genetic testing, surveillance gastroscopy and prophylactic gastrectomy are recommended. In response, at the 2004 meeting of The New Zealand Familial Gastric Cancer Group (scientists, clinicians, and allied health professionals[12]) consensus guidelines were established based on collective clinical experience managing these families and the literature. At that time, there were 45 HDGC families reported worldwide, 10 from New Zealand.

In the initial 5 years after CDH1 mutations were described, several key papers were published on genetic counseling,[13] the cumulative risk of gastric and breast carcinoma,[14] prophylactic gastrectomy,[15-17] early gastric pathology,[18-20] and surveillance chromogastroscopy.[21]

In 2008, at the seventh workshop of the IGCLC, updated consensus guidelines were generated.[22] Management algorithms have been formulated highlighting the salient management decisions.[22,23] Now, there are well over 100 HDGC families reported in the literature. The information from the published pedigrees of the first 87 families reported (up to 2008) is summarized in **Table 1** including mutation details, number of gastric and breast cancers, known histotypes, age at diagnosis, and cancers at other sites.

FAMILIAL GASTRIC CANCER: EPIDEMIOLOGY, RISK ASSESSMENT, AND PENETRANCE

Familial aggregation is reported in up to 15% of stomach cancer patients,[28–30] but only around 5% of cases in low-risk countries have an autosomal dominant pattern of inheritance.[31] Only 1% to 3% of all gastric cancers are thought to be caused by an inherited cancer syndrome.[12,22] This incidence is likely to be less among populations with a high risk of gastric cancer, such as in Japan where only 0.9% of cases had an autosomal dominant pattern.[25]

Accurate assessment of risk is paramount in reaching decisions about management options in familial cancer. Explanation of risk to patients can be difficult. Although cumulative risk in populations can be described, there is "no statistical justification for the application of a population incidence to an individual."[32] When existing knowledge does not permit accurate determination of individual risk, estimates from familial cancer registries are the most reliable reference for patients who carry germline mutations.

Based on pedigree data from 11 of the first HDGC families identified, the cumulative risk estimate for advanced gastric cancer by 80 years was estimated to be 67% in men and 83% in women with wide CIs; the mean age at diagnosis was 40 years.[14] Although no firm evidence exists for variable penetrance, comparison of the penetrance data from the largest HDGC families raises this possibility. In Family A it is 70% at 60 years, whereas in the Newfoundland family it was 40% in males and 63% in females at 75 years.[2,10]

Despite that well over 100 HDGC families have been reported, the 2001 study of 11 families (including Family A) remains the only published penetrance data available to guide risk assessment (unless the patient is a member of Family A or the Newfoundland family). Unpublished, updated data presented at the seventh IGCLC meeting indicated the lifetime risk is greater than 80%.[22] It is possible that the first 11 families identified represent a cluster of HDGC families with a particularly early age of onset. Of the 80 cases of gastric cancer within these 11 families, 28 patients (35%) were from Family A, which has a relatively high penetrance at a young age.

Only 5 (6%) of the first 87 HDGC families (see **Table 1**) have a case of advanced gastric cancer diagnosed before age 20 years. Furthermore, four of these nine cases before 20 years are from Family A, the youngest was 14 years old. In 14 families (16%), the youngest affected family member was 20 to 25 years old at diagnosis. In most HDGC families, the youngest affected family member was diagnosed in the mid-to-late twenties or early thirties. In seven HDGC families (8%), all family members were greater than 50 years old when diagnosed.

This family variation affects the guidelines made regarding the age to offer genetic testing, surveillance, and prophylactic gastrectomy.[12] It is important to recognize that age-related management recommendations are guidelines only. The age of onset and penetrance information from each HDGC family should be considered and, in some HDGC families with relatively late onset, the timing of interventions may be influenced accordingly.[23,33]

GENETICS OF HDGC

There are several comprehensive articles on the genetics of HDGC that cover technical aspects of *CDH1* mutation testing, the types of mutations found, and their effect.[34–36] *CDH1* germline mutations are only detected in families with DGC and never in families with IGC.[37] The first *CDH1* founder mutation reported was from the large Newfoundland, Canada, family. In addition, haplotype analysis suggests two other families may have a common ancestor.[10] The ethnicity of HDGC families is diverse, although it is notable that only eight are from Asia. Given the high incidence of

Table 1

Germline *CDH1* mutations: details of HDGC families and early-onset, sporadic gastric cancer cases-review of published mutations as of March 2008

Family Identification	Ethnicity: Country	CDH1 Mutation	Type	Exon Intron	Mutation Effect	GC (DGC) Cases	Age of GC Cases	Mean Age	Breast (LBC)	Age of Breast Ca	Other Cancers	Reference
C7	ns: North America	3G>C	Non	1	No protein	1 (1)	73	NA	1 (1)	73	—	Suriano 2005[70]
203	European	45insT	ins	1	Truncation	4 (2)	30-67	44	1 (1)	—	3xCo (1xSRC)	Oliveira 2002[24]
—	White	49-2A>C	ss	In 1	—	4 (3)	42, 54, 57, 68	—	1	—	Cr, S, Pr, Bl, Pa, T	More 2007[71]
—	White: UK	49-2A→G	ss	in 1	truncation	6 (4)	34-69	49	nil	55	Lu, Co	Richards 1999[72]
—	ns: Irish	As above	"	"	"	2 (2)	ns	—	ns	—	—	Moran 2005[73]
C220	White	53delC	del	2	truncation	2 (2)	28-48	38	nil	—	Lu, Cx	Humar 2002[74]
—	White: UK	59G→A	non	2	truncation	3 (3)	27-50	38	nil	—	—	Richards 1999[72]
4201	White: USA	70G→T	non	2	truncation	4 (3)	37-46	42	3	39, 39, 46	Leu x2 (45, 66y)	Guilford 1999[3]
—	Japanese	185G→T	mis	3	missense	7 ?	46-72	59	nil	—	—	Shinmura 1999[25]
—	White: USA	187C>T	non	3	truncation	3 (2)	33-85	62	1	—	2x Co, Pr, ZxEn	Gayther 1998[75]
F6	North American	As above	"	"	"	3 (1)	24-52	?	3 (2)	39, 39, 56	LBC 39x2, 1 mixed ca	Suriano 2005[70]
DST	Maori: NZ	190C→T	non	3	truncation	2 (2)	22, 28 + others	?	—	?	+ 'digestive ca' at 25y	Guilford 1999[3]
—	White: French	283C→T	non	3	truncation	4 (3)	34, 42, 43, 47	?	2	64, +ns	Dussaulax 2001[76]
F1	Unknown	As above	"	"	"	7 (2)	39-76	—	nil	—	ns	Kaurah 2007[10]
F2	White	353C>G	mis	3	missense	2 (1)	55, 63	—	nil	—	—	More 2007[71]
—	White: German	372delC	del	3	truncation	4 (2)	15, 37, 38, 58	37	1 (1)	49	—	Keller 1999[77]
F10	Italian	382delC	del	3	—	7 (1)	32, 40, 42, 45, 50, 55, 56	46	2	—	—	Brooks-Wilson 2004[26]
—	White	531+2T>A	ss	In4	truncation	5 (3)	36, 53, 48, 22, 23	—	1	43	4xcleft lip or palate	Frebourg 2006[78]
RS	White: France	586G→T	non	5	truncation	4 (4)	31-55	45	nil	—	—	Guilford 1999[3]
F1	Northern European	687(+1)G>A	ss	Int 5	—	4 (1)	36, 40, 48, 50	43	1	—	—	Brooks-Wilson 2004[26]
—	Caucasian	715G>A	Mis,ss	6	missense	2 (2)	30, 29	—	nil	—	1 mutation +ve alive at 79	More 2007[71]
F2	Filipino	As above	"	"	"	4 (1)	29-33	—	nil	—	—	Karurah 2007[79]
G2	Korean	731A→G	mis	6	missense	7 ?	?38-63	?	nil	—	—	Yoon 1999[80]
215	Finnish	808T>G	mis	6	missense	1	Late 70s	—	nil	—	HPC: 4xPr in 70s	Ikonen 2001[81]
195	Pakistani	832G→A	ss	6	truncation	10 (6)	23-70	37	1	37	—	Oliviera 2002[82]

Family	Population	Mutation	Type	Exon/Intron	Effect	n (affected)	Age(s)				Other features	Reference
F26	Northern European	892G→A	mis	7	missense	3 (2)	32, 33, 36	34	—	—	—	Brooks-Wilson 2004[26]
23	Swedish	1003C→T	Non	7	truncation	3 (2)	22, 44, 45	—	1 (0)	51 ductal	Pr x1 86y	Jonsson 2002[83]
F1	North American	As above	"	"	"	8 (2)	25–67	—	nil	—	ns	Suriano 2005[70]
F3	North American	As above	"	7	truncation	5 (1)	35–55	—	nil	—	ns	Suriano 2005[70]
A	Maori: NZ	1008G→T	ss	7	truncation	28 (9)	14–74	33	2 (1)	Bi lob 43, 49	Co	Guilford 1998[2]
185	European	1018A>G	mis	8	missense	2	35–47	39	—	—	Ovary	Oliviera 2002[82]
F25	Northern European	1064insT	ins	8	—	3 (2)	34, 50, 58	47	Nil	—	—	Brooks-Wilson 2004[26]
—	Hispanic	1107delC	del	8	Truncation	3 (2)	27, 48, ?	—	Nil	—	—	More 2007[71]
—	Italian	1118C>T	mis	8	Missense	3 (3)	70, 72, 79	—	nil	—	Co x 1	Roviello 2007[84]
F41	Spanish	1134del8ins5	Del-in	8	—	4 (3)	27, 30, 32 +[b]	—	nil	—	—	Brooks-Wil 2004[26]
SF1	Italian: Brazil	1137G>A	ss	8	ns	3 (2)	18, 28, 37	—	nil	—	Cleft palate, aplasia cutis, partial acrania	Frebourg 2006[78]
F5	White	As above	"	8	"	1 (1)[b]	ns[b]	—	Unknown	—	—	More 2007[71]
F6	White: Swiss	As above	"	"	"	1 (1)	29	—	1	69	Saliv gland 26y, Co, 2x bilateral lung	More 2007[71]
F3a	unknown	As above	"	"	"	7 (1)	26–44	—	1	—	—	Kaurah 2007[10]
F4a	Sweden or Norway	As above	'	"	"	3 (2)	37–48	—	nil	—	—	Kaurah 2007[10]
chg72	African American	1137+1G→A	ss	Int 8	truncation	5 (4)	25–58	42	4	—	—	Guilford 1999[3]
F9	Northern European	1212delC	del	9	—	5 (4)	17, 32, 46, 47, 61	41	—	—	SRC colon	Brooks-Wilson 2004[26]
F7	Northern European	1226T→C	mis	9	missense	1 (1)	51	51	—	—	—	Brooks-Wilson 2004[26]
—	Japanese	1243A>C	mis	9	missense	5 (2)	60–63	62	—	—	—	Wang 2003[85]
—	White	1397-92delTC	Del	10	truncation	2 (2)	34, 61	—	1	78	—	More 2007[71]
F5	English	1460T→C	mis	10	missense	4 (2)	31–82	—	1	62	—	Kaurah 2007[10]
G1001	Korean	1472-73insA	ins	10	truncation	2 ?	? 42–49	—	nil	—	—	Yoon 1999[80]
PQ036	European	1476delAG	Del	10	truncation	3 (2)	32–40	35	—	—	—	Oliviera 2002[82]
F18	Northern European	1507C>T	non	10	Truncation	2 (1)	32–40	36	nil	—	—	Brooks-Wilson 2004[26]
—	Chinese	—	—	—	—	ns (1)	—	—	1 (1)	—	Proband DGC and LBC	Jiang 2004[86]
C230	Arab	1565+1G→T	ss	Int 10	truncation	3 (2)	49–56	52	nil	—	—	Humar 2002[74]
1000	White: USA	1588insC	ins	11	truncation	3 (3)	40–63	50	1	—	—	Guilford 1999[3]

(continued on next page)

Table 1 (continued)

Family Identification	Ethnicity: Country	CDH1 Mutation	Type	Exon Intron	Mutation Effect	GC (DGC) GC Cases	Age of GC Cases	Mean Age	Breast (LBC)	Age of Breast Ca	Other Cancers	Reference
—	Spanish	1610delC	del	11	truncation	3 (3)	50, 58, 71	—	1 (1)	<50y	Pr, Co	Rodriguez 2006[87]
—	European or German	1619insG	ins	11	—	1 (1)	29	29	1	49, bilat	Ab, Lu	Keller 2004[88]
F6	Irish	1682insA	ins	11	—	3 (1)	38-52	—	1 (1)	38y + DGC	Note 38y DGC & LBC	Kaurah 2007[10]
C210	African American	1710delT	del	11	truncation	2 (2)	19, 29	24	1	—	Pr	Humar 2002[74]
—	White: USA	1711 insG	Ins	11	truncation	9 ?	30-68	45	nil	—	—	Gayther 1998[75]
F11	Northern European	1711 + 5G>A	ss	In11	—	3 (3)	44-48	45	5 (1)	—	—	Brooks-Wilson 2004[26]
HPc31	Sweden	1774G>A	mis	12	unknown	2	69, 85	—	2	46, 54 (1-ve)	Pr x4 (mean age 69) 1xCo	Jonsson 2002[83]
F2	Northern European	1779insC	Ins	12	—	3 (3)	33-42	37	—	—	—	Brooks-Wilson 2004[26]
—	White: Canada	1792C→T	Non	12	truncation	6 (3)	23-43	31	—	—	—	Gayther 1998[75]
C200	Maori: NZ	As above	"	"	"	3 (1) ?	30-41	35	—	—	Pan	Humor 2002[74]
F5	North America	As above	"	"	"	4 (1)	30-54	—	2	—	—	Suriano 2005[70]
SF2[a]	Portuguese	1901C→T	mis	12	missense	1 (1)	30	-	nil	—	—	Suriano2003[27]
32SF[a]	Portuguese	As above	"	"	"	2	23, 26	—	nil	—	—	Oliviera 2004[89]
F7	English: no linkage	As above	"	"	"	2 (1)	34, 45	—	1	75	—	Kaurah 2007[10]
F8	Maori	As above	"	"	"	2 (2)	25, 30s	—	nil	—	—	More 2007[71]
F8	Spanish	1913G>A	Non	12	ns	10 (1)	21-59	—	nil	—	—	Kaurah 2007[10]
16, SF4	Northern European	2061delTG	del	13	—	2 (2)	24, 47	36	nil	—	—	Brooks 04+Kaurah
SF9	English or Scottish	As above	"	"	"	3 (1)	37-80	—	2	65?	—	Kaurah 2007[10]
C	Maori: NZ	2095C→T	non	13	truncation	ns	ns	ns	—	—	—	Guilford 1998[2]
P9	Chinese	As above	"	"	"	3 (3)	24, 39, 55	—	—	—	—	More 2007[71]
F9	North American	2161C>G	ss	13	—	4 (1)	21-75	—	nil	—	—	Suriano 2005[70]
F10	Unavailable	2164 + 5G>A	ss	In13	—	3 (1)	38-44	—	nil	—	—	Kaurah 2007[10]
F13sf5	Northern European	2195G→A	mis	14	missense	2 (2)	36-70	53	4 (2)	44-86	Note br ca both families	Brooks 04+Kaurah
F11	English: no linkage	As above	"	"	"	3 (2)	32-65	—	4 (1)	40-77	Note br ca both families	Kaurah 2007[10]
F12	Colombian	2245C>T	mis	14	Missense	3 (2)	36-49	—	nil	—	—	Kaurah 2007[10]
F2	North American	2276delG	del	14	—	10 (2)	35-87	—	2 (1)	—	—	Suriano 2005[70]

Family	Ethnicity	Mutation	Type	Exon/Intron	Effect	No. DGC (families)	Age	Age	No. LBC (families)	Age	Other cancers	Reference
240	White	2295 + 5G→A	ss	Int 14	truncation	4 (2)	44–52	47	nil	—	—	Humar 2002[74]
F4	Northern European	2310delC	Del	15	—	8 (≥1)	42–79[b]	61[b]	1	—	—	Brooks-Wilson 2004[26]
HPC	Swedish	2329G>A	mis	15	n.s	1	74	—	nil	—	Pr x 3 (mean 68y)	Jonsson 2002[83]
F13	English	2343A>T	mis	15	—	2 (2)	51, 63	—	1	ns	—	Kaurah 2007[10]
B	Maori: NZ	2381insC	ins	15	truncation	7 (2)	30 (16–35)[b]	30[b]	ns	—	—	Guilford 1998[2]
—	German	2396C→G	mis	15	—	3 (1m)	41–52[b]	47[b]	—	—	—	Keller 2004[88]
SF6, 7 F14,15	Newfoundland founder mutation	2398delC	del	15	ns	29 (7)	25–80	—	16 (4)	41–68	Cox8, Leux3, head or neck2, My, Lu, Br, Es, NHL,	Kaurah 2007[10]
—	Japanese	2494G→A	mis	16	missense	7 (1)	ns	ns	—	—	—	Yabuta 2002[90]
—	White	2440-6C>G	ss	In 15	—	2 (2)	36, ns	—	nil	—	Lu	More 2007[71]
—	Summary	87 families 68 mutations	—	—	30% miss 70% trun	—	5 with case <20, 9 with case <20–24	—	75 (18)	Youngest case 38y	—	—
Solitary Cases												
—	European: Canada	41delT	del	1	—	1 (1)	30	—	—	—	—	Bacani 2006[91]
C5	North American	1063 del 6	del	8	Truncation	1 (1)	27	—	—	—	—	Suriano 2005[70]
C6	North American	1285 C>T	mis	9	missense	1 (1)	27	—	—	—	—	Suriano 2005[70]
MFW	Not specified	1487del7	del	10	truncation	1 (1)	31	—	—	—	Father: co at 60y	Guilford 1999[3]
g71	African American	1849G→A	mis	12	missense	1	64	—	—	—	—	Ascano 2001[92]
293	African American	1849G→A	mis	12	missense	1	43	—	—	—	Not related to 294	Suriano 2003[27]
294	African American	1849G→A	mis	12	missense	1	43	—	—	—	Not related to 293	Suriano 2003[27]
Breast Cancer Family												
LBC	USA	517insA	ins	4	truncation	nil	—	—	2 (2)	28, 42	Melanomax2, kidney	Masciari 2007[93]

Abbreviations: DGC, diffuse gastric cancer; GC, gastric cancer; LBC, lobular breast cancer; Mutation type: del, deletion; del-in, deletion-insertion; ins, insertion; mis, missense; non, nonsense; ss, splice site; Other cancers: Ab, abdominal; Bl, bladder; Br, breast; Co, colorectal; Cx, cervix; En, endometrium; Es, esophagus; HPC, hereditary prostate cancer; Lu, lung; Leu, leukemia; Ly, lymphoma; mis, missence; My, myeloma; NHL, non-Hodgkins Lymphoma; ns, not stated; Ov, ovary; Pan, pancreas; Pr, prostate; SRC, signet ring cell; T, testicular.

[a] Haplotype analysis suggests common ancestor.

[b] Age of ≥1 case of GC not known.

sporadic gastric cancer in Asian populations, chance clusters of sporadic gastric cancer may obscure the identification of families with inherited susceptibility.

Germline *CDH1* mutations are spread relatively evenly throughout the gene, with 70% truncating and 30% missense mutations. Although truncating mutations clearly abrogate normal E-cadherin function, the functional significance of missense mutations is not straightforward. Cell aggregation and invasion assays have been developed to evaluate the effect of *CDH1* missense mutations.[27,38] When combined with other parameters, missense mutations can be classified as a "silent polymorphism, variant of uncertain significance, or likely deleterious variant"[22] to guide genetic counseling.

Five germline *CDH1* mutations have been identified in eight unrelated cases of young-onset, sporadic, gastric cancer. Given the absence of a family history of cancer in these individuals, these rare isolated cases are likely to represent de novo or low penetrance *CDH1* mutations.[39]

PATHOLOGY OF HDGC

The hallmark of early HDGC is the presence of multiple foci of signet ring cell carcinoma (SRCC) confined to the superficial lamina propria—TNM stage T1a (**Fig. 1**) with no nodal metastases.[15,19,20] HDGC prophylactic gastrectomy specimens nearly always appear macroscopically normal as the microscopic early HDGC foci typically

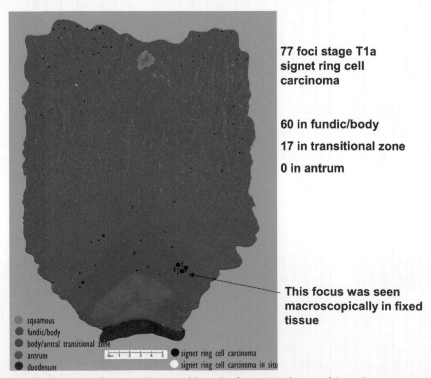

77 foci stage T1a signet ring cell carcinoma

60 in fundic/body

17 in transitional zone

0 in antrum

This focus was seen macroscopically in fixed tissue

squamous
fundic/body
body/antral transitional zone
antrum
duodenum

signet ring cell carcinoma
signet ring cell carcinoma in situ

Fig. 1. Gastrectomy from a 28-year-old male from Family A subjected to a research pathology mapping protocol. After fixation, a 10 mm confluent pale area was evident, which corresponded to a cluster of foci of SRCC (*arrow*), the 3 largest were 3–5 mm. Total number of HDGC foci was 77. At surveillance chromogastroscopy, two pale areas were seen in the proximal antrum, greater curve. One biopsy of each area was taken: both SRCC.

lie beneath an intact surface epithelium with no visible alteration to pit pattern. However, complete pathologic mapping of these specimens as part of a research protocol reveals a wide variation in the number of T1a foci (range 1–487, **Table 2**). Only one stomach mapped in this detailed fashion had no foci of carcinoma identified.[12,18,19,22]

Carneiro and colleagues[18] first described in situ signet ring cells (SRCs) and page-toid spread of SRCs below preserved epithelium of glands and foveolae in HDGC stomachs. Whether these are actual precursor lesions of the T1a invasive foci or are markers of E-cadherin insufficiency within the epithelial cells as they migrate up toward the gastric lumen is likely a moot point. Both of these possibilities have been raised in the two proposed models of HDGC.[18,42]

Pathologic mapping of the 19 gastrectomy specimens from New Zealand families revealed there is a greater density of foci (which are typically larger) in the transitional zone between body and antral type mucosa and the antrum is usually spared.[12,19,23,40] This has ramifications for endoscopic screening but it should be noted that this pattern has not been detected in the other HDGC mapping studies.[18,41] Given that 16 stomachs are from Family A, a genotype-phenotype correlation is possible.

In advanced stages, HDGC is indistinguishable from advanced, sporadic DGC. In HDGC gastrectomy series (see **Table 2**), the average age is 32 years and the presence of T1a carcinoma in all (100%) stomachs contrasts markedly with the estimated penetrance for advanced HDGC at the same age, which is 4%.[14] Even allowing for an extended time lag for progression from these early HDGC foci, the penetrance for advanced HDGC at 50 years is still only 21% in men and 46% in women.[14] These observations suggest that a prolonged indolent phase may occur before stage T1a HDGC foci invade beyond the mucosa; however, the duration of this indolent phase remains unpredictable.[12]

MODELS OF HDGC

The existence of multiple microscopic foci of early (stage T1a) SRCC with reduced E-cadherin expression in the stomachs of germline *CDH1* mutation carriers strongly suggests that E-cadherin deficiency can initiate carcinogenesis and, in HDGC, is not an event associated with late-stage invasion and metastasis. The development of SRCC in *cdh1*± mice supports this, as does the finding of allele-specific monoclonal *CDH1* promoter methylation in T1a foci from human mutation carriers.[42] These results provide compelling evidence for a tumor suppressor role of E-cadherin in diffuse gastric carcinogenesis.

Although the concept that E-cadherin loss alone can initiate gastric cancer of SRC phenotype may seem logical given that *CDH1* mutation causes HDGC, this is not definitively proven. Despite this, it is clear that E-cadherin loss is at least an early event of importance before invasion of muscle layers and metastasis. Given that the many hundreds of human T1a foci display E-cadherin downregulation, it seems highly unlikely that any gene other than *CDH1* is consistently mutated.

Drawing on research in *cdh1*± mice and *CDH1* mutation carriers, the author, working with others, has proposed a model for the initiation of gastric SRCC.[43,44] E-cadherin downregulation is believed to be the initiating event. Consistent with the cancer stem cell hypothesis, evidence suggests this occurs in the gastric stem cell and/or progenitor cells, which are thought to be located in upper isthmus of the neck of the gastric glands.[44]

How altered E-cadherin mediated cell-to-cell adhesion actually initiates cancer is not known. It has been hypothesized that it "disrupts the integrity of the epithelial

Table 2
HDGC case series: pathologic mapping of gastrectomies

Case Series	Average Number of Blocks per Stomach	Average Number of Sections per Stomach	Mutation Family ID	Age: Sex	Number of Foci	Mean Foci per Stomach (Average Age)
NZ Series[40]	200 (range 153–284)	453 (range 286–548)	1008 G → T Family A	15 cases		118 foci (33y)
—	—	—	1792 C → T	43 f	4	n.a
—	—	—	2287 G → T	33 f	32	n.a
—	—	—	1792 C → T	63 M	26	n.a
North American Series[20]	not stated (range 68–258)	each block contains ≥1 sections (exact number not stated)	1588insC Family 3	41 f	13	16 foci (40y)
				39 m	2	
				37 f	5	
				47 f	15	
				40 m	45	
—	—	—	1792 C → T Family 1	35 f	55	n.a
—	—	—	1711 insG Family 2	40 m	3	2 foci (23y)
				22 m	2	
				28 f	1	
Stanford Series[41]	118 (range 99–156)	118 One per block	1003 C → T	53 f	17	14 foci (53y)
				52 f	16	
				55 f	17	
				50 f	15	
				56 m	4	
				51 m	13	
—	—	—	2395 del C	42 f	2	n.a
—	—	—	1565 + 2ins T	70 f	3	n.a

monolayer or promotes division of cells away from the epithelial plane,"[43] possibly related to disorientation of the mitotic spindle' - a concept illustrated in Guilford and colleagues.[43] In this situation the progenitor cell could either end up just beneath the basement membrane in the lamina propria or be shed into the lumen. If lying beneath the basemant membrane, the cancer stem cell or progenitor cell then proceeds as if It were still within the epithelium- it divides and produces daughter cells. If the daughter cells are programmed to differentiate along the mucous neck cell lineage, the result will be classical SRCs—full of mucous. The classical SRCs end up lying beneath the normal surface epithelium. Over time, the cancer stem-cell progenitor may accumulate more genetic errors and gain the capacity to invade beyond the T1a stage: the progression phase of carcinogenesis. This seems to be associated with SRC activation and acquisition of poor differentiation.[44]

The early HDGC neoplastic lesion is relatively hypoproliferative compared with the adjacent epithelium with a lower expression of the Ki67 proliferation marker than the surrounding nonmalignant tissues.[44] This is in stark contrast to the usual perceptions of initiating events in cancer involving a hyperproliferative state caused by mutations in genes implicated in cell cycle control or cell survival. The disruption of these processes early in carcinoma initiation is supported by the functions of many of the known cancer susceptibility genes, for example *APC*, *SMAD4*, *P53*, *BRCA1/2*, *MET*, *PTCH*, or *CDKN2A*.[42]

Diagnosis

Gastric cancer families can present when a family member is newly diagnosed with gastric cancer or a patient, concerned about family history, requests screening. These patients should be referred to their local Clinical Genetics Service for evaluation and counseling. Depending on the assessed risk, genetic testing may be appropriate. The diagnosis of HDGC was approached in two slightly different ways in the literature. Initially, in 1999, Guilford and colleagues[3] proposed that HDGC was defined genetically by E-cadherin mutation carriage. That same year the IGCLC proposed clinical criteria for HDGC,[11] which is now commonly applied. Awareness of this difference is important clinically because management recommendations differ dependending on if a mutation is identified or not.

Obviously, risk is more easily quantified when a *CDH1* mutation is detected. In contrast, when a family qualifies for *CDH1* mutation testing and no mutation is found or a mutation of indeterminate significance is identified, the situation is more complex with little evidence to guide best practice. Dealing with uncertainty is difficult and stressful for patients. The care of all patients meeting clinical criteria for HDGC is enhanced by involvement of a multidisciplinary team. Ideally, this should occur early on so that a management strategy that is appropriately tailored to the risk evident from the family pedigree can be developed.

CDH1 GENETIC TESTING AND MUTATION SEARCHING

Informed consent and genetic counseling are fundamental in familial cancer protocols. The American Society of Clinical Oncology recommends that an individual should not be tested for a cancer predisposition gene unless there is a reasonably high likelihood of detecting a disease causing mutation and the result is intended to influence medical management.[45] In the diagnosis of familial gastric cancer, once histotype is known, the next step is to see if the family history fits the newly agreed on, broader, IGCLC criteria (see later discussion). In families with IGC and those with DGC not meeting criteria for *CDH1* mutation testing, the only genetic testing available is under the auspices of research for new mutations in candidate genes.

The original IGCLC criteria were (1) two confirmed cases of DGC in first-degree or second-degree relatives with the diagnosis in one made under age 50 years or (2) three confirmed cases of DGC at any age. These criteria were relaxed because it is often not possible to confirm histotype in more than one family member.[26] Testing of families meeting these criteria will reveal a *CDH1* mutation in 30% to 50% of cases.[24,26]

Searching for *CDH1* mutations in young-onset, sporadic, DGC patients is controversial because of the low mutation yield, averaging 7% (range 0%–20%) across eight studies.[33] Testing has been suggested if an individual with DGC is younger than 35 years or, alternatively, 45 years of age.[26,27] The IGCLC recently settled on 40 years of age.[22] An additional criteria for testing has been suggested: a family or personal history of DGC and lobular breast cancer if one member is younger than 50 years.[22,26]

MINIMUM AGE FOR GENETIC TESTING AND INTERVENTIONS IN HDGC

Many factors need to be considered when counseling HDGC families before testing children and adolescents. These include psychological impact, informed consent, the limitations of surveillance techniques, and the morbidity and mortality of prophylactic gastrectomy. Probably the most important is age-related risk. The risk of advanced HDGC in children is very low and, using the data of Pharoah and colleagues,[14] it can be estimated to be less than 1% at age 20 years, rising to 4% at age 30 years.

The world-view on predictive genetic testing in children and adolescence is underpinned by the philosophies of nonmalevolence and autonomy.[46] Previously, genetic testing was only performed in situations in which there was clear benefit to the child or adolescent through surveillance or medical intervention. More recently, as collective experience widened, this view has been challenged, acknowledging that many of the previously held concerns, although valid, were theoretical and did not allow for the possible benefits of testing.[47] These include providing time for parents and children to adjust to future risks and the removal of uncertainty. Findings suggest that most children do not suffer clinically significant psychological distress as a direct result of genetic testing.[48,49]

Acknowledging the child as part of the family and moving toward a family-centered approach is central to this issue.[50] Recognizing individual family members' autonomy continues to be an important principle in this approach and it remains the responsibility of the health professional to determine if an adolescent is competent to participate in the genetic counseling process and make an informed choice. Studies in this area have used genetic testing in familial adenomatous polyposis as a model.[48,51,52] Although this model has merit, there are important differences between it and HDGC, including the penetrance and the consequences of total colectomy versus total gastrectomy.

The consensus in New Zealand is that usually genetic testing for *CDH1* mutation should not be offered until 16 years of age. However, the testing of HDGC family members 14 to16 years of age should be reviewed on a case-by-case basis, taking into account factors such as the maturity of the child, the anxiety expressed by both child and family, and the individual family history. To the author's knowledge, testing below age 14 years of age has only occurred once in a family when a death had occurred from gastric cancer in a 14-year-old child and the parents wanted their three children tested at the same time. Acknowledging that countries have slightly differing legislation on age limits for consent, the latest IGCLC guidelines recommends testing can begin "from the age of consent (16/18y)."[22]

SURVEILLANCE AND SCREENING GASTROSCOPY IN HDGC

By definition, mutation carriers have surveillance gastroscopy and screening is taking place when no mutation has been detected or mutation testing is not indicated. Gastroscopy is the only technique currently considered a possible surveillance or screening measure for individuals with a high risk of gastric cancer. There are no clinical trials on which to base recommendations for surveillance or screening in HDGC. From 1999 to 2003, an observational study in HDGC was conducted. It followed 33 CDH1 mutation carriers from New Zealand and used annual chromoendoscopy, a technique no longer performed.[21]

The role of gastroscopy in HDGC is somewhat problematical because of the inherent limitations of trying to reliably detect early DGC, which typically infiltrates beneath an intact surface epithelium without producing ulceration or elevation of the mucosa. Consistent with this, in nearly all prophylactic gastrectomies, despite normal preoperative endoscopy, microscopic foci of early HDGC are identified; albeit in most cases the foci are smaller than 3 mm. It would be difficult to detect foci this tiny with white light endoscopy.

Despite concerns about the low sensitivity of gastroscopy in early detection of HDGC foci, gastroscopy has a role in the management of familial gastric cancer. Clinicians must ensure their patients understand these limitations and the potential consequence. In New Zealand, patients are advised that "an unquantifiable risk exists that a gastric cancer can be missed on gastroscopy, even at advanced stages."[53] At each annual endoscopy, it is reiterated that prophylactic gastrectomy is the only way to reliably remove the risk of death from gastric cancer.

When prophylactic gastrectomy is declined or deferred, the onus is on the clinician to establish the patient's reasons for this decision and to make sure the patient has adequate understanding, making their decision an informed choice. This discussion takes time and it is key that the multidisciplinary team is involved.

The indications for screening gastroscopy include (1) HDGC patients in whom no mutation has been detected and (2) patients with a family history of intestinal type gastric cancer. The indications for surveillance in CDH1 mutation carriers include (1) work-up before prophylactic gastrectomy (baseline endoscopy), (2) patients who decline prophylactic surgery or are not fit for surgery, (3) patients with CDH1 mutations of indeterminate significance, (4) patients wishing to temporarily defer prophylactic surgery, and (5) when mutation testing is performed younger than the usual recommended age (ie, below age 16) and the timing of prophylactic surgery is deferred.

The New Zealand consensus is that surveillance gastroscopy is an acceptable option up to age 20 years and that prophylactic gastrectomy is not usually recommended younger than this age.[12] In general, surveillance gastroscopy is poorly tolerated in children less than 14 years of age, despite presenting few difficulties in older age groups. Between ages 14 to 16 years, gastroscopy should be considered on a case-by-case basis.

Endoscopy Technique

In 1999, the IGCLC initially recommended a "thorough 30-minute endoscopy, every 6 months by a team experienced at diagnosing early gastric cancer." In New Zealand, in the first 5 years after genetic testing began (1999–2003), the 33 mutation carriers identified refused prophylactic gastrectomy. The gastroenterologist at Tauranga Hospital,

David Shaw, did a literature search on methods to enhance detection of early gastric cancer. A trial of chromogastroscopy using congo red and methylene blue dyes was performed in an effort to improve the sensitivity of detection of early HDGC.

Experience from the initial 5 years of annual chromogastroscopy in Family A showed chromoendoscopy was an improvement over standard white light gastroscopy, facilitating detection of 56 "pale lesions" in 10 patients, of which 23(41%) were carcinoma. The pale lesions were 3 to 10 mm, with those highly suspicious for carcinoma having distinct pallor.[21] Correlation with the HDGC pathologic mapping study showed biopsied lesions correspond to the larger foci (4–10 mm) and that lesions smaller than 4 mm were not readily detected by chromogastroscopy.

Chromoendoscopy was discontinued in New Zealand in 2005 because of concerns over congo red toxicity. Subsequently, the two gastroenterologists regularly performing the HDGC endoscopies began detecting pale lesions on standard white light endoscopy with biopsy proving carcinoma (David Shaw, Susan Parry, personal communication, 2009–2011). The experience with chromoendoscopy led to an appreciation that pale areas are visible at standard endoscopy. However, they are so subtle they would easily be overlooked as within normal limits by most endoscopists. In all New Zealand HDGC patients in whom carcinoma has been diagnosed at surveillance, the biopsied pale areas were located in the transitional zone area or immediately adjacent to it, irrespective of whether the biopsy was chromo or white light directed.

The IGCLC recommends a protocol of multiple random biopsies. This has not been the approach in the New Zealand HDGC surveillance program. Multiple random gastric biopsies taken during surveillance gastroscopy usually fail to detect carcinoma in HDGC.[15,18,20] The rationale behind the New Zealand approach is that evidence shows occult tiny early HDGC foci exist in almost all HDGC gastrectomies when examined using a detailed research protocol. Patients are advised their stomachs will almost certainly contain microscopic early SRC cancer irrespective of a normal appearance at endoscopy. If random biopsies are undertaken, the detection of a cancer focus becomes a chance event, which means patients selection for gastrectomy is somewhat akin to a lottery. The opposing argument in favor of random biopsies is based on the premise that random biopsies are more likely to be positive in HDGC stomachs with a higher number of foci of early cancer. The problem with this assumption is that there is no evidence that a higher number of foci in a mutation carriers stomach corresponds to a greater likelihood of developing advanced gastric cancer. Although this is an understandable assumption, all foci are at the same stage.

Reliable detection of tiny HDGC foci (smaller than approximately 4 mm) anywhere in the stomach is possibly an unrealistic expectation by standard white light techniques. Although newer endoscopic modalities (eg, narrow band, confocal imaging) may help, perhaps a better approach is to find a selective marker that optically enhances SRCs and not normal tissue (or visa versa). This could be a labeled marker injected before endoscopy or, alternatively, a technology that exploits the difference in naturally occurring fluorescence properties between malignant and normal tissue.

TOTAL GASTRECTOMY IN HDGC

The indications for gastrectomy in HDGC are either with prophylactic intent or therapeutic when carcinoma is detected at surveillance. Before prophylactic gastrectomy, a baseline endoscopy should be undertaken—usually no sign of malignancy is evident. However, given almost all HDGC stomachs harbor occult foci of SRCC, it could be argued all gastrectomies in HDGC are, strictly speaking, therapeutic because it is known that foci of SRCC will be present if looked for hard enough. The issues surrounding prophylactic surgery in HDGC are covered in detail in the 2008 IGCLC consensus guidelines[22] and are reviewed in several case series.[12,15,17]

It is widely agreed that surgery should be strongly considered once a mutation has been detected.[22] In adult mutation carriers, a strong recommendation is, in many respects, easier to explain and justify and the approach advocated in New Zealand that gastrectomy should be advised in all mutation carriers older than 20 years of age has been endorsed by the IGCLC.[22] However, the exact timing of prophylactic surgery if testing is done in the early teenage years is not established and represents a complex clinical scenario requiring careful consideration and balancing of risks.

Mortality and Morbidity Risks

Patients need to be fully informed of the mortality risk and long-term consequences of total gastrectomy. In the twenty-first century, the issues surrounding prophylactic total gastrectomy relate more to its lifelong morbidities than the mortality risk, although the latter cannot be overlooked. The practice in New Zealand is to quote a risk of less than 1% for fit young mutation carriers although, when performed in a specialist, high-volume, upper-gastrointestinal unit, it is likely to be less than this.[54] The mortality in most recent series ranges from 0% to 6%.[17,55] However, most patients in these series are elderly. In recent years there has been a decline in perioperative mortality after major gastrointestinal surgery due to advances in surgical technique, anesthesia, and intensive care.

Total gastrectomy results in lifelong vitamin B12 deficiency and predisposes to iron malabsorption and deficiency. Roux-en-Y reconstruction means food bypasses the duodenum and a variable length of proximal jejunum, which are the major sites for vitamin D, iron, folate, and calcium absorption. Decreased intestinal transit time is thought to cause a degree of fat malabsorption in most patients, reducing absorption of vitamins A, D, E, and K. Although the increased risk of osteoporosis, osteomalacia, and malnutrition after gastrectomy is well described in gastric cancer patients, usually aged 60 to 70 years,[56] there is little data on the risk in younger age.

The need for altered meal size, frequency, and content can considerably affect lifestyle. This needs full discussion, as does the nature of dumping syndrome and the nutritional consequences, including the need for life-long vitamin B12 injections. Input from a dietician is essential in the care of these patients.

Staging and Technical Aspects

Patients with surveillance-detected gastric carcinoma should be staged in the same manner as sporadic gastric malignancy with CT scanning and, if appropriate, an endoscopic ultrasound. In New Zealand, in therapeutic total gastrectomy for sporadic gastric cancer, D2 dissection with preservation of spleen and pancreas is the standard operative approach, which is likewise applied to HDGC patients with surveillance-detected cancer. In contrast, with the prophylactic gastrectomy cases, a D1 dissection is performed by most surgeons in New Zealand in line with IGCLC guidelines.[22]

The controversy surrounding the increased mortality risk versus survival benefit in D2 versus D1 resection for gastric cancer has been subject to extensive review and is covered elsewhere this issue in articles by Hoshi and Hundahl.[57] Evidence suggests that, when performed in specialist, upper-gastrointestinal units, D2 resection without resection of spleen or distal pancreas confers little, if any, additional risk and would generally be performed in HDGC patients with surveillance-detected cancer.[12,15,19,20,23] However, to the author's knowledge, no nodal metastases have been reported in a therapeutic gastrectomy in early HDGC. However, this is a small group of patients, most from the New Zealand series. Because of the stealth-like characteristics of advanced DGC, it is not impossible that preoperative staging investigations will understage HDGC patients. In the future, it may become evident that modified D2 gastrectomy is not necessary in selected HDGC patients with surveillance-detected cancer; however, until that time, the consensus in New Zealand is in favor of modified D2 dissection.[23]

Roux-en-Y esophagojejunostomy reconstruction without construction of a jejunal pouch reservoir is the standard approach.[12,17] Although there is some evidence that a jejunal pouch leads to improved food intake and weight gain in the early postoperative months, the long-term benefits have previously been considered marginal,[55] although a recent randomized trial looking at the benefit of Roux-en-Y pouch reconstruction suggests some long-term benefit.[58]

It is essential to ensure the complete resection of the gastric mucosa. There is no palpable or visible serosal surface marking indicating the squamocolumnar gastroesophageal junction (GEJ). In New Zealand, the esophagus is transected 3 to 4 cm above the anatomic junction and an intact cuff of squamous esophageal mucosa is visually confirmed via an incision at the apex of the fundus.[12] Lewis and colleagues[17] comment that, despite initial transection 2 cm above the apparent anatomic GEJ, gastric mucosa remained at the esophageal margin, necessitating additional resection in two patients. They advocate intraoperative gastroscopy to identify the GEJ and suggest intraoperative frozen section is mandatory to confirm the margin. Management of the gastroduodenal junction is easier because the palpable pyloric sphincter provides a reliable indication of the mucosal transition but, again, New Zealand practice is to visually confirm an intact rim of duodenal mucosa.[12]

Prognosis and Follow-Up After Gastrectomy

Survival data from early gastric cancer series provide an indication of likely prognosis in early HDGC. Five-year survival is over 90% in almost all Western and Japanese early gastric cancer series and, in T1a lesions, approaches 95%.[59] The general clinical perception is that SRCC and diffuse gastric carcinoma per se confer a worse prognosis than the intestinal type.[60] However, stage-for-stage survival from gastric SRCC is similar[61] or, for early diffuse type, significantly better than other types.[62–64] This is illustrated by a large Korean series that compared 263 early gastric SRCCs with 670 early non-SRC cancers: 5-year survival was 94% and 92%, respectively, and 10-year survival was 90% and 79%.[62]

Consequently, if HDGC foci are limited to the gastric mucosa, prognosis is likely to be excellent following total gastrectomy. It is possible that gastrectomies curative for gastric disease will unmask an additional risk of carcinoma at other sites in HDGC patients. There is no indication for follow-up gastroscopy after gastrectomy unless symptoms develop. Follow-up should include review of nutrition, weight, B12 injections and other supplement intake, and bone health, including possible bone density testing.

Management Approach in Teenage Years

Gastrectomy is associated with a reduction in body weight, often exceeding 10%,[55,56] and is likely to compromise growth in teenagers. By the age of 18 years in boys and 15 years in girls, 97% have finished height growth and weight increase begins to level off.[65] Prophylactic gastrectomy is not usually recommended in mutation carriers under 20 years of age. The rational is that, broadly, the risk of a CDH1 mutation carrier developing advanced gastric cancer before the age of 20 years (<1%) is approximately matched by the mortality risk of prophylactic total gastrectomy in this age group. Seven members of family A have had therapeutic gastrectomy at age 15 to 19 years, all diagnosed at surveillance gastroscopy.

Fertility issues
Given that the pelvic cavity is not disturbed by gastrectomy, and providing there are no major postoperative complications, a significant reduction in female fecundity is unlikely. Data is limited to anecdote: women have successfully carried to full-term after total gastrectomy for HDGC in the United Kingdom[22] and New Zealand. The nutritional consequences of gastrectomy theoretically may affect in utero growth and nutrition but, again, data is limited. After gastrectomy, all women should seek nutritional advice before conception. Although it seems unlikely that a decision to have a total gastrectomy would compromise a woman's future fertility, this possibility should be discussed.[12]

Managing risk of lobular breast cancer and other malignancies
The preliminary estimated cumulative risk of breast cancer in HDGC is 39% (95% CI, 12%–84%) at 80 years of age.[14] In the large Canadian HDGC family with 16 cases of breast cancer (ages 41–68 years) estimated cumulative risk was 52% (95% CI, 29%–94%) by 75 years of age. Molecular and histologic studies on sporadic breast cancer support the association between HDGC and infiltrating lobular carcinoma.[9,66]

Lobular breast cancer is more difficult to detect by mammography than the ductal type because of its diffuse growth pattern and relative lack of microcalcification. MRI is more sensitive, although along with this goes a higher rate of false positives.[67,68] Regular breast examination by a specialist is an essential part of any surveillance program. Taking the lead from protocols used in BRCA mutation carriers, 6 monthly breast examinations and a yearly interval for radiological surveillance would seem appropriate beginning at age 35 years. Routine prophylactic mastectomy is not recommended, but may be appropriate some families.[23]

Colorectal, prostate, and other cancers have been documented in HDGC families, but not at frequencies significantly above the risk of the general population. SRC carcinoma of the colon has been reported in HDGC families.[24,26] At present there is no evidence to justify surveillance of other organs over and above that recommended in population-based cancer screening programs.

Helicobacter pylori eradication, lifestyle advice, and chemoprevention
If Helicobacter pylori is present it should be eradicated.[12,22] H pylori infection does not seem to play a major role in HDGC[15,19,20]; however, it is possible it may modify disease risk.[16] It would seem appropriate that surveillance is accompanied by general lifestyle advice about known risk factors for sporadic gastric cancer, such as reducing intake of salted, cured, and preserved foods; increasing intake of fresh fruit and vegetables; not smoking; and avoiding excessive alcohol.[69] There are no trials of chemoprevention in HDGC. A trial of chemoprevention in a murine model of HDGC with a cyclooxygenase (COX)-2 inhibitor and chlorophyllin did not suggest any benefit.[40]

SUMMARY

HDGC is a challenging familial cancer syndrome to manage. Surveillance endoscopy is far from a fail-safe technique. No long-term observational or randomized trial data exist. The ideal surveillance modality would exploit the duration of the indolent phase of HDGC, allowing gastrectomy to take place if and/or when T1a foci begin invading the muscularis mucosae. Given the diffuse morphologically of this type of gastric cancer, it will likely prove very difficult to develop a surveillance modality that reliably detects early progression. Currently, the only way to eliminate the risk of gastric cancer is prophylactic total gastrectomy—a procedure with significant risks to life and health.

The management of HDGC has advanced dramatically in 14 years since *CDH1* mutations were described. This has involved international collaboration between many research groups around the world. Clinicians in New Zealand, a small remote country with only 4 million people, had to grapple early on with the management of 10 HDGC families, including Family A, the original and largest known HDGC family. Over 120 members of Family A have undergone genetic testing and 50 mutation carriers have been identified. The approach to counseling, genetic testing, surveillance, and surgery described has achieved wide acceptance in New Zealand HDGC families. In the words of one family member, "the nightmare is nearly over."

ACKNOWLEDGMENTS

Thank you to Dr Amanda Charlton, Pathologist, University of Auckland, New Zealand, who reported the gastrectomy slides and produced this **Fig. 1**.

REFERENCES

1. Lugli A, Zlobec I, Singer G, et al. Napoleon Bonaparte's gastric cancer: a clinicopathologic approach to staging, pathogenesis, and etiology. Nat Clin Pract Gastroenterol Hepatol 2007;4:52.
2. Guilford P, Hopkins J, Harraway J, et al. E-cadherin germline mutations in familial gastric cancer. Nature 1998;392:402.
3. Guilford P, Hopkins J, Grady W, et al. E-cadherin germline mutations define an inherited cancer syndrome dominated by diffuse gastric cancer. Hum Mutat 1999;14:249.
4. Jones E. Familial gastric cancer. N Z Med J 1964;63:287.
5. Lauren P. The two histological main types of gastric carcinoma: diffuse and so-called intestinal-type carcinoma. Acta Pathol Microbiol Scand 1965;64:31.
6. Shimoyama Y, Hirohashi S. Expression of E- and P-cadherin in gastric carcinomas. Cancer Res 1991;51:2185.
7. Becker K, Atkinson M, Reich U, et al. E-cadherin gene mutations provide clues to diffuse type gastric carcinomas. Cancer Res 1994;54:3845.
8. Machado JC, Soares P, Carneiro F, et al. E-cadherin gene mutations provide a genetic basis for the phenotypic divergence of mixed gastric carcinomas. Lab Invest 1999;79:459.
9. Chan J, Wong C. Loss of E-cadherin is the fundamental defect in diffuse-type gastric cancer and infiltrating lobular carcinoma of the breast. Adv Anat Pathol 2001;8:165.
10. Kaurah P, MacMillan A, Boyd N, et al. Founder and recurrent CDH1 mutations in families with hereditary diffuse gastric cancer. JAMA 2007;297:2360.
11. Caldas C, Carneiro F, Lynch HT, et al. Familial gastric cancer: overview and guidelines for management. J Med Genet 1999;36:873.
12. Blair V, Martin I, Shaw D, et al. Hereditary diffuse gastric cancer: diagnosis and management. Clin Gastroenterol Hepatol 2006;4:262–75.
13. Lynch HT, Grady W, Lynch JF, et al. E-cadherin mutation-based genetic counseling and hereditary diffuse gastric carcinoma. Cancer Genet Cytogenet 2000;122:1.
14. Pharoah P, Guilford P, Caldas C, et al. Incidence of gastric cancer and breast cancer in CDH1 (E-cadherin) mutation carriers from hereditary diffuse gastric cancer families. Gastroenterology 2001;121:1348.

15. Chun YS, Lindor NM, Smyrk TC, et al. Germline E-cadherin mutations: is prophylactic gastrectomy indicated? Cancer 2001;92:181.
16. Fitzgerald RC, Caldas C. Clinical implications of E-cadherin associated hereditary diffuse gastric cancer. Gut 2004;53:775.
17. Lewis FR, Mellinger JD, Hayashi A, et al. Prophylactic total gastrectomy for familial cancer. Surgery 2001;130:612.
18. Carneiro F, Huntsman DG, Smyrk TC, et al. Model of the early development of diffuse gastric cancer in E-cadherin mutation carriers and its implications for patient screening. J Pathol 2004;203:681.
19. Charlton A, Blair V, Shaw D, et al. Hereditary diffuse gastric cancer: predominance of multiple foci of signet ring cell carcinoma in distal stomach and transitional zone. Gut 2004;53:814.
20. Huntsman DG, Carneiro F, Lewis FR, et al. Early gastric cancer in young asymptomatic carriers of germline E-cadherin mutations. N Engl J Med 2001;344:1904.
21. Shaw D, Blair V, Framp A, et al. Chromoendoscopic surveillance in hereditary diffuse gastric cancer: an alternative to prophylactic gastrectomy? Gut 2005;54:461.
22. Fitzgerald R, Hardwick R, Huntsman D, et al. Hereditary diffuse gastric cancer: updated consensus guidelines for clinical management and directions for future research. J Med Genet 2010;47:436.
23. Blair V, Parry S. Familial gastric cancer. In: Clark S, editor. A guide to cancer genetics in clinical practice. Shrewsbury (United Kingdom): TFM Publishing Ltd; 2008.
24. Oliveira C, Bordin MC, Grehan N, et al. Screening E-cadherin in gastric cancer families reveals germline mutations only in hereditary diffuse gastric cancer kindred. Human Mutation 2002;19:510.
25. Shinmura K, Kohno T, Takahashi M, et al. Familial gastric cancer: clinicopathological characteristics, RER phenotype and germline p53 and E-cadherin mutations. Carcinogenesis 1999;20:1127.
26. Brooks-Wilson AR, Kaurah P, Suriano G, et al. Germline E-cadherin mutations in hereditary diffuse gastric cancer: assessment of 42 new families and review of genetic screening criteria. J Med Genet 2004;41:508.
27. Suriano G, Oliveira C, Ferreira P, et al. Identification of CDH-1 germline missense mutations associated with functional inactivation of the E-cadherin protein in young gastric cancer probands. Hum Mol Genet 2003;12:575.
28. La Vecchia C, Negri E, Franceschi S, et al. Family history and the risk of stomach and colorectal cancer. Cancer 1992;70:50.
29. Park JG, Yang HK, Kim WH, et al. Report on the first meeting of the international collaborative group on hereditary gastric cancer. J Natl Cancer Inst 2000;92:1781.
30. Zanghieri G, Di Gregorio C, Sacchetti C, et al. Familial occurrence of gastric cancer in the 2-year experience of a population-based registry. Cancer 1990;66:2047.
31. Kjartansson I, Jonsson Eldon B, Arinbjarnarson S, et al. Genetic epidemiologic aspects of gastric cancer in Iceland. J Am Coll Surg 2002;195:181.
32. Furnival C. Relevant risk for women with BRCA1 and BRCA2 mutations. ANZ J Surg 2007;77:309.
33. Pedrazzani C, Corso G, Marrelli D, et al. E-cadherin and hereditary diffuse gastric cancer. Surgery 2007;142:645.
34. Barber M, Murrell A, Ito Y, et al. Mechanisms and sequelae of E-cadherin silencing in hereditary diffuse gastric cancer. J Pathol 2008;216:295.

35. Oliveira C, Seruca R, Carneiro F. Genetics, pathology and clinics of familial gastric cancer. Int J Surg Pathol 2006;14:21.
36. Schrader K, Huntsman D. Hereditary diffuse gastric cancer. Cancer Genet 2010; 155:33.
37. Guilford PJ, Blair V, More H, et al. A short guide to hereditary diffuse gastric cancer. Hered Cancer Clin Pract 2007;5:183.
38. Suriano G, Seixas S, Rocha J, et al. A model to infer the pathogenic significance of CDH1 germline missense variants. J Med Genet 2006;84:1023–31.
39. Jarvinen HJ. Genetic testing for polyposis: practical and ethical aspects. Gut 2003;52:ii19.
40. Blair VR. Hereditary diffuse gastric cancer: of mice and man, in department of surgery. Auckland (New Zealand): University of Auckland; 2009.
41. Rogers W, Dobo E, Norton J, et al. Risk-reducing total gastrectomy for germline mutations in E-cadherin (CDH1): pathologic findings with clinical implications. Am J Surg Pathol 2008;32:799.
42. Humar B, Blair V, Charlton A, et al. E-cadherin deficiency initiates gastric signet-ring cell carcinoma in mice and man. Cancer Res 2009;69(5):2050–6.
43. Guilford P, Humar B, Blair V. Hereditary diffuse gastric cancer: translation of CDH1 germline mutations into clinical practice. Gastric Cancer 2010;13(1): 1–10.
44. Humar B, Fukuzawa R, Blair V, et al. Destabilized adhesion in the gastric proliferative zone and c-Src kinase activation mark the development of early diffuse gastric cancer. Cancer Res 2007;67:2480.
45. Statement of American Society of Clinical Oncology: genetic testing for cancer susceptibility. J Clin Oncol 1996;14:1730.
46. Clarke A. Clinical Genetics Society: the genetic testing of children: report of a working party of the Clinical Genetics Society (A Clarke, chairman). J Med Genet 1994;31:785.
47. Robertson S, Savulescu J. Is there a favour of predictive genetic testing in young children? Bioethics 2001;15:26.
48. Codori AM, Zawacki KL, Petersen GM, et al. Genetic testing for hereditary colorectal cancer in children: long-term psychological effects. Am J Med Genet A 2003;116:117.
49. Michie S, Bobrow M, Marteau T. Predictive genetic testing in children and adults: a study of emotional impact. J Med Genet 2001;38:519.
50. McConkie-Rosell A, Spiridigliozzi GA. "Family Matters": a conceptual framework for genetic testing in children. J Genet Couns 2004;13:9.
51. Clarke A. Parents' responses to predictive genetic testing in their children. J Med Genet 1997;34:174.
52. Michie S. Reply: parents' responses to predictive genetic testing in their children. J Med Genet 1997;34:174.
53. Shaw D, Blair V, Martin I. Chromoendoscopic surveillance in a Maori kindred genotypically predisposed to hereditary diffuse gastric cancer: an alternative to prophylactic gastrectomy [abstract: M1839]. Orlando (FL): Digestive Diseases Week; 2003.
54. Brennan M. Safety in numbers. Br J Surg 2004;91:653.
55. Lehnert T, Buhl K. Techniques of reconstruction after total gastrectomy for cancer. Br J Surg 2004;91:528.
56. Liedman B. Symptoms after total gastrectomy on food intake, body composition, bone metabolism and quality of life in gastric cancer patients—is reconstruction of a reservoir worthwhile? Nutrition 1999;15:677.

57. McCulloch P, Nita M, Kazi H, et al. Extended versus limited lymph node dissection technique for adenocarcinoma of the stomach. Cochrane Database Syst Rev 2004;4:CD001964.
58. Fein M, Fuchs K, Thalheimer A, et al. Long-term benefits of Roux-en-Y pouch reconstruction after total gastrectomy: a randomized trial. Ann Surg 2008;247:759.
59. Everett S, Axon A. Early gastric cancer in Europe. Gut 1997;41:142.
60. Barr H, Greenall M. Carcinoma of the stomach. In: Morris PJ, Wood WC, editors, Oxford textbook of surgery, vol. 2. Oxford (UK): Oxford University Press; 2000. p. 1313.
61. Kim JP, Kim SC, Yang HK. Prognostic significance of signet ring cell carcinoma of the stomach. Surg Oncol 1994;3:221.
62. Hyung WJ, Noh SH, Lee JH, et al. Early gastric carcinoma with signet ring cell histology. Cancer 2002;94:78.
63. Maehara Y, Sakaguchi Y, Moriguchi S, et al. Signet ring cell carcinoma of the stomach. Cancer 1991;69:1645.
64. Otsuji E, Yamaguchi T, Sawai K, et al. Characterization of signet ring cell carcinoma of the stomach. J Surg Oncol 1998;67:216.
65. Penfold J. Growth and its abnormalities. In: Robinson MJ, Roberton DM, editors. Practical paediatrics. 3rd edition. London (UK): Churchill Livingstone; 1994. p. 507.
66. Berx G, Van Roy F. The E-cadherin/catenin complex: an important gatekeeper in breast cancer tumorigenesis and malignant progression. Breast Cancer Res 2001;3:289.
67. Kriege M, Brekelmans C, Boetes C, et al. Efficacy of MRI and mammography for breast-cancer screening in women with a familial or genetic predisposition. N Engl J Med 2004;351:427.
68. Leach M, Boggis C, Dixon A, et al. Screening with magnetic resonance imaging and mammography of a UK population at high familial risk of breast cancer: a prospective multicentre cohort study (MARIBS). Lancet 2005;365:1769.
69. Kelley JR, Duggan JM. Gastric cancer epidemiology and risk factors. J Clin Epidemiol 2003;56:1.
70. Suriano G, Yew S, Ferreira P, et al. Characterisation of a recurrent germ line mutation of the E-cadherin Gene: Implications for genetic testing and clinical management. Human Cancer Biology 2005;11(15):5401–9.
71. More H, Humar B, Weber W, et al. Identification of seven novel germline mutations in the human E-cadherin (CDH1) gene. Human Mutation 2007;28(2):203–11.
72. Richards FM, McKee SA, Rajpar MH, et al. Germline E-cadherin gene (CDH1) mutations predispose to familial gastric cancer and colorectal cancer. Human Molecular Genetics 1999;8(4):607–10.
73. Moran CJ, Joyce M, McAnena OJ. CDH1 associated gastric cancer: a report of a family and review of the literature [review]. European Journal of Surgical Oncology 2005;31(3):259–64.
74. Humar B, Toro T, Graziano F, et al. Novel germline CDH1 mutations in hereditary diffuse gastric cancer families. Human Mutation 2002;19(5):518–25.
75. Gayther SA, Gorringe KL, Ramus SJ, et al. Identification of germ-line E-cadherin mutations in gastric cancer families of European origin. Cancer Research 1998;58(18):4086–9.
76. Dussaulx-Garin L, Blayau M, Pagenault M, et al. A new mutation of E-cadherin gene in familial gastric linitis plastica cancer with extra-digestive dissemination. Eur J Gastroenterol Hepatol 2001;13:711–5.

77. Keller G, Vogelsang H, Becker I, et al. Diffuse type gastric and lobular breast carcinoma in a familial gastric cancer patient with an E-cadherin germline mutation. American Journal of Pathology 1999;155(2):337–42.
78. Frebourg T, Oliveira C, Hochain P, et al. Cleft lip/palate and CDH1/E-cadherin mutations in families with hereditary diffuse gastric cancer. Journal of Medical Genetics 2006;43(2):138–42.
79. Kaurah P, MacMillan A, Boyd N, et al. Founder and recurrent CDH1 mutations in families with hereditary diffuse gastric cancer. JAMA 2007;297(21):2360–72.
80. Yoon K, Ku J, Yang H, et al. Germline mutations of E-cadherin gene in Korean familial gastric cancer patients. J Hum Genet 1999;44:177–80.
81. Ikonen T, Matikainen M, Mononen N, et al. Association of E-cadherin germ-line alterations with prostate cancer. Clin Cancer Res 2001;7(11):3465–71.
82. Oliveira C, Bordin MC, Grehan N, et al. Screening E-cadherin in gastric cancer families reveals germline mutations only in Hereditary Diffuse Gastric Cancer kindred. Human Mutation 2002;19(5):510–7.
83. Jonsson BA, Bergh A, Stattin P, et al. Germline mutations in E-cadherin do not explain association of hereditary prostate cancer, gastric cancer and breast cancer. Int J Cancer 2002;98(6):838–43.
84. Roviello F, Corso G, Pedrazzani C, et al. Hereditary diffuse gastric cancer and E-cadherin: description of the first germline mutation in an Italian family. European Journal of Surgical Oncology 2007;33(4):448–51.
85. Wang HD, Ren J, Zhang L. CDH1 germline mutation in hereditary gastric carcinoma. World J Gastroenterol 2004;10:3088–93.
86. Jiang Y, Wan YL, Wang ZJ, et al. Germline E-cadherin gene mutation screening in familial gastric cancer kindreds. Chinese Journal of Surgery 2004;42(15):914–7 [in Chinese].
87. Rodriguez-Sanjuan JC, Fontalba A, Mayorga M, et al. A novel mutation in the E-cadherin gene in the first family with hereditary diffuse gastric cancer reported in Spain. European Journal of Surgical Oncology 2006;32:1110–3.
88. Keller G, Vogelsang H, Becker I, et al. Germline mutations of the E-cadherin(CDH1) and TP53 genes, rather than of RUNX3 and HPP1, contribute to genetic predisposition in German gastric cancer patients. J Med Genet 2004;41(6):e89.
89. Oliveira C, Ferreira P, Nabais S, et al. E-Cadherin (CDH1) and p53 rather than SMAD4 and Caspase-10 germline mutations contribute to genetic predisposition in Portuguese gastric cancer patients. European Journal of Cancer 2004;40(12):1897–903.
90. Yabuta T, Shinmura K, Tani M, et al. E-cadherin gene variants in gastric cancer families whose probands are diagnosed with diffuse gastric cancer. Int J Cancer 2002;101(5):434–41.
91. Bacani JT, Soares M, Zwingerman R, et al. CDH1/E-cadherin germline mutations in early-onset gastric cancer. Journal of Medical Genetics 2006;43(11):867–72.
92. Ascano JJ, Frierson H Jr, Moskaluk CA, et al. Inactivation of the E-cadherin gene in sporadic diffuse-type gastric cancer. Modern Pathology 2001;14(10):942–9.
93. Masciari S, Larsson N, Senz J, et al. Germline E-cadherin mutations in familial lobular breast cancer. Journal of Medical Genetics 2007;44(11):726–31.

Standard D2 and Modified Nodal Dissection for Gastric Adenocarcinoma

Hisakazu Hoshi, MD

KEYWORDS

- Gastric cancer • Stomach cancer • Surgical technique
- D2 nodal dissection

D2 nodal dissection for the treatment of a gastric cancer was initially proposed by a Japanese surgeon, Tamaki Kajitani, in 1942 when the long-term result of surgical resection carried poor prognosis for this disease. Since then, numerous studies of lymphatic pathways have been performed and nodal stations around the stomach defined. In 1962, the first edition of the Japanese Classification of Gastric Cancer was published by the Japanese Research Society for Gastric Cancer (JRSGC), which defined the classifications and rules for the treatment of gastric cancer. In Japan, this was widely accepted and operations were standardized for the location of the primary lesion and the stage of the disease. Originally, the D2 nodal dissection, which removes all the first-tier and second-tier nodal stations, was recommended for all stages of gastric cancer. In recent years, these recommendations have been modified for early gastric cancer.[1]

The extent of the nodal dissection for gastric adenocarcinoma has been a topic of debate for a few decades. The most recent update of the Dutch D2 - D1 trial showed improved locoregional disease control in the D2 group but failed to show improvement in overall survival.[2] The study was criticized for underdissection or overdissection of the nodal stations as well as the high morbidity/mortality associated with the pancreatosplenectomy, which canceled out any potential survival benefit of the D2 nodal dissection. The surgical quality control and the learning curve on an unfamiliar procedure proved to be a major difficulty in a surgical trial (see the articles by Sasako and Hundahl elsewhere in this issue).

Intuitively, the groups of patients with gastric cancer who receive maximum potential benefit from the D2 nodal dissection are those with stage Ib to IIIa by the American Joint Committee on Cancer (AJCC) Cancer Staging Manual, seventh edition.[3] In 2004,

---

The author has nothing to disclose.
Surgical Oncology and Endocrine Surgery, Department of Surgery, University of Iowa Hospitals and Clinics, 200 Hawkins Drive, 4637 JCP, Iowa City, IA 52242, USA
E-mail address: hisakazu-hoshi@uiowa.edu

Surg Oncol Clin N Am 21 (2012) 57–70
doi:10.1016/j.soc.2011.09.004
1055-3207/12/$ – see front matter © 2012 Elsevier Inc. All rights reserved.

the Japanese Gastric Cancer Association (JGCA, formerly the JRSGC) published the second edition of the gastric cancer guideline and defined the modified nodal dissections.[1] In 2010, refinements and simplifications of the previous guidelines were put forth based on published nodal metastasis data from the National Cancer Center and Cancer Research Institute in Japan.[4] Since then, patients with early gastric cancer (stage Ia) are offered minimally invasive gastrectomies with modified nodal dissections in Japan. This article discusses the anatomy and the exposure of the nodal basins (stations) necessary to perform D2 nodal dissection, modifications to the standard nodal dissection based on tumor location and stage, and the difficulties presented by these demanding procedures.

DEFINITION OF THE NODAL STATIONS AND THE D1 AND D2 NODAL DISSECTIONS

The nodal stations around the stomach are anatomically defined and numerically classified by the Japanese Classification of Gastric Carcinoma published by JGCA (**Fig. 1**, **Table 1**).[5] Perigastric nodal stations are numbered 1 to 6 and regional nodal stations are 7 to 12. Nodal stations numbered higher than 12 are generally considered distant nodal stations and are not dissected for the standard D2 nodal dissection, except nodal station 14v (discussed later).

The level of the nodal dissection, known as the D number, is defined by the guidelines from JGCA.[4] Although the classic D1 nodal dissection is defined by complete dissection of the first-tier nodal stations, which are determined by the location of the primary lesion, and is most compatible with the current concept of the D1 nodes, perigastric nodes (station 1–6) in Western literature, the current (2010) definition of D1 nodal dissection in Japan includes the left gastric artery node station (station 7) in addition to the perigastric nodal stations because of the observed high rate of metastasis in this nodal station by early gastric cancer.

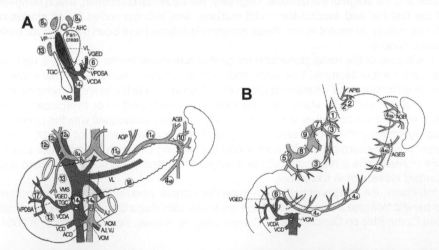

Fig. 1. (*A, B*). Location and border of lymph node stations by the JGCA. ACM, *A. colica media*; AGB, *Aa. gastricae breves*; AGES, *A. gastroepiploica sinistra*; AGP, *A. gastrica posterior*; AHC, *A. hepatica communis*; AJ, *A. jejunalis*; APIS, *A. phrenica inferior sinistra*; TGC, *Truncus gastrocolicus*; VCD, *V. colica dextra*; VCDA, *V.colica dextra accessoria*; VCM, *V. colica media*; VGED, *V. gastroepiploica dextra*; VJ, *V. jejunalis*; VL, *V. lienalis*; VMS, *V. mesenterica superior*; VP, *V. portae*; VPDSA, *V. pancreaticoduodenalis superior anterior*; (*From* Japanese Gastric Cancer Association. Japanese classifications of gastric carcinoma. 14th edition. Tokyo (Japan): Kanehara & Co; p. 14, 15; with permission.)

Table 1
Anatomic definitions of lymph node (LN) stations

No.	Definition
1	Right paracardial LNs, including those along the first branch of the ascending limb of the left gastric artery
2	Left paracardial LNs including those along the esophagocardiac branch of the left subphrenic artery
3a	Lesser curvature LNs along the branches of the left gastric artery
3b	Lesser curvature LNs along the second branch and distal part of the right gastric artery
4sa	Left greater curvature LNs along the short gastric arteries (perigastric area)
4sb	Left greater curvature LNs along the left gastroepiploic artery (perigastric area)
4d	Right greater curvature LNs along the second branch and distal part of the right gastroepiploic artery
5	Suprapyloric LNs along the first branch and proximal part of the right gastric artery
6	Infrapyloric LNs along the first branch and proximal part of the right gastroepiploic artery down to the confluence of the right gastroepiploic vein and the anterior superior pancreatoduodenal vein
7	LNs along the trunk of the left gastric artery between its root and the origin of its ascending branch
8a	Anterosuperior LNs along the common hepatic artery
8p	Posterior LNs along the common hepatic artery
9	Celiac artery LNs
10	Splenic hilar LNs including those adjacent to the splenic artery distal to the pancreatic tail, and those on the roots of the short gastric arteries and along the left gastroepiploic artery proximal to its first gastric branch
11p	Proximal splenic artery LNs from its origin to halfway between its origin and the pancreatic tail end
11d	Distal splenic artery LNs from halfway between its origin and the pancreatic tail end to the end of the pancreatic tail
12a	Hepatoduodenal ligament LNs along the proper hepatic artery, in the caudal half between the confluence of the right and left hepatic ducts and the upper border of the pancreas
12b	Hepatoduodenal ligament LNs along the bile duct, in the caudal half between the confluence of the right and left hepatic ducts and the upper border of the pancreas
12p	Hepatoduodenal ligament LNs along the portal vein in the caudal half between the confluence of the right and left hepatic ducts and the upper border of the pancreas
13	LNs on the posterior surface of the pancreatic head cranial to the duodenal papilla
14v	LNs along the superior mesenteric vein
15	LNs along the middle colic vessels
16a1	Para-aortic LNs in the diaphragmatic aortic hiatus
16a2	Para-aortic LNs between the upper margin of the origin of the celiac artery and the lower border of the left renal vein
16b1	Para-aortic LNs between the lower border of the left renal vein and the upper border of the origin of the inferior mesenteric artery
16b2	Para-aortic LNs between the upper border of the origin of the inferior mesenteric artery and the aortic bifurcation

(continued on next page)

Table 1 (continued)	
No.	Definition
17	LNs on the anterior surface of the pancreatic head beneath the pancreatic sheath
18	LNs along the inferior border of the pancreatic body
19	Infradiaphragmatic LNs predominantly along the subphrenic artery
20	Paraesophageal LNs in the diaphragmatic esophageal hiatus
110	Paraesophageal LNs in the lower thorax
111	Supradiaphragmatic LNs separate from the esophagus
112	Posterior mediastinal LNs separate from the esophagus and the esophageal hiatus

Data from Japanese Gastric Cancer Association. Japanese classifications of gastric carcinoma. 14th edition. Tokyo (Japan): Kanehara & Co Ltd.

THE TECHNIQUE OF D2 NODAL DISSECTION (DISTAL AND TOTAL GASTRECTOMY)

Typically, a D2 nodal dissection starts from the greater curvature of the stomach. An omentectomy is an integral part of the D2 nodal dissection. The lesser sac is accessed by detaching the greater omentum from the transverse colon. Once it is widely separated then the greater omentum can be seen to be fused with the anterior surface of the transverse colon mesentery on the right side (**Fig. 2**). This portion is considered right side border of the lesser sac. Access to station 6 (the infrapyloric nodal station) is gained by further separating the omentum from the transverse colon mesentery by dividing this right side border peritoneum (see **Fig. 2** yellow line). Once they are completely separated then the middle colic vessels and a right accessory colic vein can be seen (**Fig 3**). By tracing the middle colic vessels, the anterior surface of the superior mesenteric vein (SMV) can be reached. The soft tissue covering the anterior surface of the SMV below the lower edge of the pancreas is classified as station 14v. If the tumor is located in the antrum of the stomach, then this station may be included in the resection (discussed later). The right accessory colic vein is located in the right side of the transverse colon mesentery, this joins with the right gastroepiploic vein, and the venous drainage from the pancreatic head then forms a gastrocolic trunk.

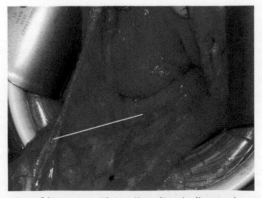

Fig. 2. Right side border of lesser sac. The yellow line indicates the peritoneal incision to further separate the greater omentum and the transverse colon mesentery.

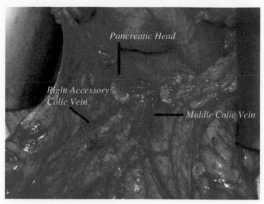

Fig. 3. Middle colic vein and right accessory colic vein.

This large vein then drains directly into the SMV (**Fig. 4**).[6] The right accessory vein is sometimes called an accessory middle colic vein; however, this article follows the JGCA and uses the term right accessory colic vein. Nodal station 6 is located proximal to the junction of the right accessory colic vein and the right gastroepiploic vein. For complete dissection of station 6, the right gastroepiploic vein should be ligated at this junction. All the soft tissues covering the anterior surface of the pancreas head are then dissected off toward the pylorus. About 5 mm to 1 cm cephalad to the right gastroepiploic vein, a right gastroepiploic artery can be seen emerging from the pancreatic head parenchyma (**Fig. 5**). This artery is ligated at this portion and all the soft tissue are cleared from the pancreas toward the inferior wall of the duodenum, which concludes the infrapyloric portion of the dissection.

At the lesser curvature of the stomach, the lesser omentum is incised along the attachment about 1 cm from the liver. The incision extends up to the esophageal hiatus. An accessory (or replaced) left hepatic artery should be recognized in the area, if present. It can be preserved by dissecting all the surrounding soft tissues if the gastric cancer is early and has a low chance of involvement of the left gastric nodes. On the left side of a hepatoduodenal ligament, soft tissue covering the proper hepatic artery is dissected toward the common hepatic artery (station 12a). As the dissection progresses toward the common hepatic artery, the origin of the right gastric artery can be seen, and this is ligated at the origin and the suprapyloric portion of the soft tissue along this artery (station 5) is separated from the hepatoduodenal ligament and head of the pancreas toward the superior duodenal wall.

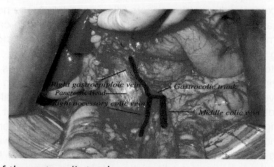

Fig. 4. Anatomy of the gastrocolic trunk.

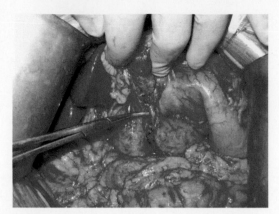

Fig. 5. Right gastroepiploic artery.

A retroperitoneal dissection can be performed without transecting the duodenum but exposure is usually better after the transection. The retroperitoneal dissection starts as a continuation of the previous proper hepatic artery node dissection. The peritoneum is divided along the superior border of the pancreas to the left and the soft tissue covering the common hepatic artery (station 8a) is dissected away. There is a distinctive plane between the nodal tissue and the pancreas parenchyma; this should be recognized and the dissection should be maintained in this plane to avoid injury to the pancreas. There are multiple small vessels present between these nodes and upper border of the pancreas and these should be recognized and coagulated before transection. The dissection plane can also be maintained just outside the perivascular nerve plexus unless gross metastatic nodes present along the artery. The left gastric vein is typically present around the common hepatic artery but may be located in front of the common hepatic artery.[7,8] Injury to this vein, often referred to as the coronary vein, creates a bleeding situation that is difficult to control. Careful dissection and vessel control before division is recommended. The superior border of the dissection is the right crus of the diaphragm.

Once the origin of the left gastric artery is identified, the soft tissue surrounding the artery is dissected distally and the vessel is ligated at the origin. After dividing the left gastric artery, the dissection proceeds along the splenic artery. About 40% to 97% of patients have a posterior gastric artery supplying the posterior portion of the gastric fundus that arises from the middle portion of the splenic artery.[9,10] Nodal tissue proximal to the origin of the posterior gastric artery (station 11p) should be dissected for all gastric cancers except early gastric cancers (discussed later). The nodal tissue distal to the posterior gastric artery (station 11d) should be dissected in cases that require a total gastrectomy. This portion of the dissection is easier after mobilization of the fundus by ligating short gastric arteries for the total gastrectomy.

In the retroperitoneum, the border of the right diaphragmatic crus is identified and peritoneum covering the crus is divided (**Fig. 6** yellow arrows), which provides access to the space between the anterior surface of the aorta and the nodal tissue along the lesser curvature of the stomach. Dissection of this plane from right to left mobilizes node stations 1 (right cardiac), 3 (lesser curvature), 7 (left gastric artery), and 9 (celiac) toward the stomach. The left side of the esophageal hiatus will eventually be completely exposed and the dissection plane should connect to the previous left gastric artery and the splenic artery dissection plane (**Fig. 7**).

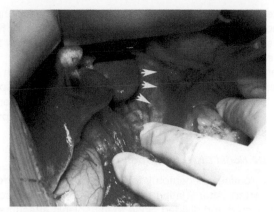

Fig. 6. Upper border of retroperitoneal dissection. Yellow arrows point out the retroperitoneal incision line along the right diaphragmatic crus.

At the greater curvature side, separation of the greater omentum from the transverse colon continues to the splenic flexure. Caution should be exercised not to pull the greater omentum to expose this area to avoid splenic capsular tears until the lower pole of the spleen is completely separated from the specimen. At the lower pole of the spleen and the tail of the pancreas, the origin of the left gastroepiploic artery and vein can be identified and these should be ligated at this point to completely clear the left greater curvature nodal tissue (station 4sb).

Completion of the D2 Nodal Dissection (Distal Gastrectomy)

In distal gastrectomy, both the lesser curvature and greater curvature of the stomach need to be cleared of nodal tissue for transection. Along the greater curvature, all the terminal branches from the left gastroepiploic artery should be ligated on the wall of the stomach starting from the first branch of the left gastroepiploic artery to the planned transection point. Preserved short gastric arteries can prevent gastric remnant necrosis if distal gastrectomy is to be performed.

On the lesser curvature, the previously dissected nodal packet needs to be separated from the stomach wall. This separation can be accomplished by ligating the

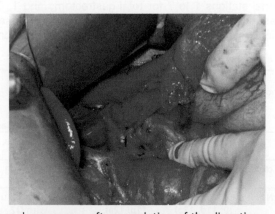

Fig. 7. Retroperitoneal appearance after completion of the dissection.

left gastric artery terminal branches on the gastric wall from the esophagogastric junction to the transection point or vice versa. The left gastric artery has anterior and posterior branches that terminate on the corresponding surfaces of the stomach, so both branches need to be ligated.

Once this portion of the dissection is completed, then the stomach should be ready to be divided to remove all the nodal tissue en bloc with the main specimen. For the clean and complete dissection of the nodes in the correct plane, en bloc resection of the celiac nodes is recommended, although left gastric artery preservation may be required for a replaced left hepatic artery.

Completion of the D2 Nodal Dissection (Total Gastrectomy)

In total gastrectomy, routine splenectomy for nodal clearance is currently not recommended (discussed later). After ligating the left gastroepiploic vessels, short gastric vessels need to be ligated and divided close to the splenic attachment. Nodal tissue located in the gastrosplenic ligament is classified as station 4sa. Once the short gastric vessels are ligated and divided, the gastric fundus can be mobilized completely from the retroperitoneum and spleen and nodal tissues along the distal splenic artery (station 11d) and the hilum of the spleen (station 10) are dissected. To avoid injury to the splenic vessels and tail of the pancreas, the dissection should follow the previous dissection plane identified at the celiac axis. The esophagus is encircled and both anterior and posterior vagus nerves are divided. All nodal tissue can now be removed en bloc with the stomach by dividing the esophagus.

INDICATION FOR MODIFICATIONS OF THE D2 NODAL DISSECTION

As discussed previously, the D2 nodal dissection is recommended for gastric adenocarcinoma of stage Ib or higher (higher than cT2 or cN1). If the depth of the tumor is either Tis or T1, then omission of certain nodal stations is considered to be acceptable (**Table 2**).

For Tis (mucosal) cancer, an endoscopic mucosal resection (EMR) or an endoscopic submucosal dissection (ESD) can be considered. Any mucosal lesion other than differentiated histology with size less than 2 cm without ulceration should be approached with caution by the endoscopic treatment because of the lack of long-term results (discussed further by Inoue and Gerke elsewhere in this issue). Mucosal cancer that cannot be treated with EMR or ESD requires currently defined D1 nodal dissection, which includes nodal stations 1 to 7 for total gastrectomy and 1, 3, 4sb, 4d, 5, 6, and 7 for distal gastrectomy (**Fig. 8**A, B). A proximal gastric mucosal cancer can be treated with proximal gastrectomy with D1 nodal dissection (stations 1, 2, 3a, 4sa,

Table 2 Modifications of nodal dissection by T stages and procedures			
	Total Gastrectomy	Distal Gastrectomy	Proximal Gastrectomy
cTis (mucosal)	D1 (1–7)	D1 (1, 3, 4sb, 4d, 5, 6, 7)	D1 (1, 2, 3a, 4sa, 4sb, 7)
cT1 (submucosal), cN0	D1 plus (D1 and 8a, 9, 11p)	D1 plus (D1 and 8a, 9)	D1 plus (D1 and 8a, 9, 11p)
cT2 or deeper or cN1	D2 (D1 plus and 10, 11d, 12a)	D2 (D1 plus and 11p, 12a)	Should be treated with total with D2

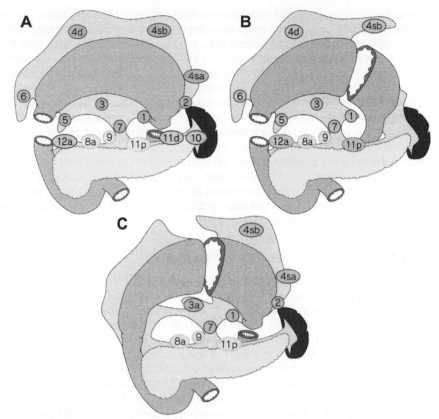

Fig. 8. Modification of nodal dissection for (*A*) total gastrectomy, (*B*) distal gastrectomy, (*C*) proximal gastrectomy. Blue nodal stations, D1; yellow nodal stations, D1 plus; red nodal stations, D2. (*From* Japanese Gastric Cancer Association. Japanese gastric cancer treatment guidelines. Tokyo (Japan): Kanehara & Co Ltd; 2010. p. 13; with permission.)

4sb, and 7). In this case, nodal stations 3b (right gastric), 4d, 5, and 6 can be omitted from the dissection (see **Fig. 8**C).

T1 (submucosal) cancer requires more than the D1 nodal dissection for adequate nodal clearance. If preoperative imaging indicates cN0 disease, then D1 plus dissection is required for a distal lesion (dissect all the D1 node plus common hepatic and celiac node [station 8a, 9]). For a lesion requiring a total gastrectomy, the D1 plus should include stations 8a, 9, and the proximal splenic nodal station (11p). cT1 with cN1 disease should be treated with the standard D2 nodal dissection as described previously.

The SMV nodal station (14v) has been a part of the D2 nodal dissection for a long time; however, the current treatment guideline by the JGCA[4] does not include this nodal station in standard D2 nodal dissection. Omission of station 14v in the guidelines is partly because of the poor prognosis associated with grossly positive 14v nodal station even when the nodal station is dissected. Because nodal stations 6 and 14v are 1 contiguous nodal structure, especially for distal gastric cancers with clinically positive infrapyloric nodes (station 6), the dissection of station 14v is recommended by many of the experts and should be considered to control micrometastatic disease until there is further evidence.

Historically, a splenectomy plus distal pancreatectomy have been an integral part of the classic D2 nodal dissection to ensure complete clearance of the splenic hilar nodal station (station 10) and the distal splenic artery nodal station (station 11d) (see the article by Hundahl elsewhere in this issue). Previous randomized trials examining D1 - D2 nodal dissection suffered from the complications of this historical approach. Currently, splenectomy and distal pancreatectomy are not recommended for nodal clearance in North America and Europe. Because of the high incidence of splenic hilar nodal involvement in advanced proximal gastric cancers, a randomized trial of D2 nodal dissections with or without a splenectomy preserving the pancreatic tail is in progress for this specific group of patients in Japan.[11]

The omentectomy is classically performed with the D2 nodal dissection but can be omitted for cTis to cT2 disease. In these cases, care should be taken to stay at least 3 cm below the gastroepiploic arcade to include all the greater curvature nodal tissue in the specimen. No randomized trial has been published to date addressing whether the omentectomy improves overall survival.

MARUYAMA INDEX AND THE D2 NODAL DISSECTION

The Maruyama Index (MI) was initially proposed by Hundahl and colleagues[12] to analyze the completeness of a nodal dissection in 2002. The computer software (WinEstimate: Jürgen Knauth, Munich, Germany) was used to predict the possibility of each nodal station involvement based on data from 4302 patients treated at the National Cancer Canter Hospital in Japan between 1968 and 1989.[13] A calculated value (MI) was used to estimate the sum of the percentages of undissected nodal stations that reflect potentially untreated disease left behind. Hundahl and colleagues[12] analyzed patients in Intergroup 0116 (SWOG 9008) and concluded that a low MI is associated with better overall survival and a MI of more than 5 is an indicator of inadequate nodal dissection. Subsequently, a similar analysis was performed on patients in the Dutch D1 - D2 trial, which confirmed the findings on a different population of the patients.[14,15]

Although the predicting model is thought to be a great tool to individually modify the extent of a nodal dissection by targeting MI less than 5, there are some issues associated with this approach. First, this prediction model requires several clinical (preoperative) data points (histology type, gross appearance of the tumor, size, and tumor depth) to run the program. Because these are preoperative data, there is a margin of error in estimation and this may call for an incorrect data set leading to either overtreatment or undertreatment. Second, an MI more than 5 needs to be interpreted with caution. High MI can occur in 2 different scenarios. One is an inadequate degree of nodal dissection and the other is advanced disease beyond the surgical treatment. The former is the case with Intergroup 0116, in which a high percentage of patients received a D0 resection. However, even in the region of the world where the D2 nodal dissection is routinely practiced, they still see high-MI cases as the disease stage advances. MI more than 5 might simply mean that the disease is too advanced to be effectively treated with the surgical measure alone. Recently, Kyong and colleagues[16] published data for distal gastric adenocarcinomas treated at the Seoul National University. They identified 1050 distal gastric adenocarcinomas treated with curative gastrectomies with extended nodal dissections in their database and calculated MI with WinEstimate. They also calculated simulated MI for the depth of each tumor treated with different levels of nodal dissection. They used the previous version of the JGCA guideline to define D1, D1plus, and D2, which are slightly different from those of the current third edition (2010) guideline.[1,4] They concluded that, to reduce the percentage of patients who have an MI more than 5, D1 plus stations 7 and 8a for mucosal cancer and D2 for submucosal or deeper should be performed. If the data are reanalyzed with current D level definitions of the JGCA guideline,[4] then the D1 nodal dissection for mucosal cancers (Tis) will produce 2.0% of patients with MI more than 5 and the D1 plus dissection will produce 0%. For submucosal tumors (T1), the D1 plus will produce 2.3% and the D2 will produce 0%. For T2 and greater, the D2 (includes 14v) will produce 2.3% for T2, 13.5% for T3, and 49.5% for T4a. If 2.3% is chosen as an acceptable cut off for patients with MI greater than 5, then the current guideline recommendation is effective and MI less than 5 can be achieved in 97.5% of patients with T2 or thinner gastric cancers without using the complicated Maruyama program (**Table 3**). For cancers of T3 and greater, because of the higher chance of extensive nodal involvement, achieving a low MI may prove more difficult especially at a time when the merits of standard D2 are still being debated.

LEARNING CURVE OF THE D2 NODAL DISSECTION AND SURGICAL QUALITY CONTROL

As previously described, D2 nodal dissection is a technically challenging procedure that calls for detailed anatomic understanding of the nodal structures around the stomach. Both UK and Dutch D1 - D2 randomized trials[17,18] suffered from high morbidity and mortality of patients in the D2 arm and underdissection of nodal stations (noncompliance). The Dutch trial had more rigorous surgical quality control than the UK trial, but they experienced an 81.5% noncompliance rate.[19]

Japanese surgical trainees typically observe a large number of D2 gastrectomy procedures early in their training. They start performing the procedure under the direct supervision of gastric cancer specialists as early as the second or third postgraduate year. Lee and colleagues[20] published the Korean experience of the learning curve on the D2 nodal dissection technique. They used node retrieval of more than 25 as a quality measure and studied 2 junior staff members who joined their National Cancer Center. Their conclusion was that at least 23 cases or 8 months of training are required to produce a 92.5% successful node retrieval rate. These 2 junior staff members were not novices and had been trained in gastric cancer surgery for 2 years at their respective university hospitals. They assisted in more than 200 gastrectomies per year before they joined the National Cancer Center and they performed gastric cancer surgery as

Table 3
Proportion of patients with MI greater than 5 in different T stage distal gastric cancer treated with current JGCA D level definition

	n	D1 (%)	D1 plus (%)	D2[a] (%)
Tis	349	7 (2.0)	0 (0)	0 (0)
T1	300	114 (38)	7 (2.3)	0 (0)
T2	130	105 (81)	31 (23.8)	3 (2.3)
T3	170	141 (83)	102 (60)	23 (13.5)
T4a	93	91 (98)	91 (97.8)	46 (49.5)
Total	1042	458 (44.0)	231 (22.2)	72 (6.9)

Data calculated by WinEstimate program.
[a] Includes 14v nodal station (see **Table 2** for detail of D level).
Data from Kong SH, Yoo MW, Kim JW, et al. Validation of limited lymphadenectomy for lower-third gastric cancer based on depth of tumour invasion. Br J Surg 2011;98(1):65–72.

first assistants for 3 months after joining. In Western institutions, it is rare to have this volume of cases and the result may not be directly applicable.

In 1996, McCulloch published his own experience of this procedure.[21] He began to perform this procedure unsupervised after spending 4 months in Japan undergoing intensive supervised training. He used physiologic score (POSSUM [Physiological and Operative Severity Score for the Enumeration of Mortality and Morbidity]) and morbidity for quality measures. His conclusion was that 18 to 24 months or 15 to 25 procedures are required to reach a plateau in learning. He did not report any changes in the number of nodal retrievals during the study period; however, the study mainly addresses the learning curve for safety, not for quality.

From the author's personal experience, to master this procedure requires some form of preparation (video instruction, assistant experience) as well as at least 20 to 30 supervised, hands-on experiences, which is difficult to achieve in most Western institutions. Furthermore, the procedure becomes technically more challenging once a patient's body mass index (BMI) exceeds 30 to 35 kg/m^2. A previous Japanese randomized D2 versus D3 trial showed that BMI greater than 25 kg/m^2 is associated with decreased nodal retrieval in D2 nodal dissection.[22] Quality control for the procedure is even more difficult in Western institutions for these reasons.

The Dutch group published surgically treated noncardia gastric cancer survival data comparing 3 different periods: the pretrial period (D1–D2 trial), the trial, and the post-trial period.[23] During the trial period, the surgical procedure for gastric cancer was standardized and surgeons were educated in the procedure. Throughout the study periods, the operative mortality remained stable from 8.4% to 5.9%. They observed statistically significant improvement in overall survival by the period once all other prognostic factors had been adjusted (**Fig. 9**). In this database, only 3 patients received chemotherapy. Even considering the improvement in perioperative care during these periods, this result is a striking reminder of the serious impact of surgical quality control on cancer treatment outcome.

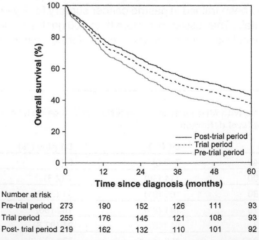

Number at risk					
Pre-trial period	273	190	152	126	111	93
Trial period	255	176	145	121	108	93
Post- trial period	219	162	132	110	101	92

Fig. 9. Overall survival of resected noncardia gastric cancer by period of diagnosis, adjusted for age, gender, tumor site, pT-stage, pN stage, and hospital volume. (*From* Krijnen P, den Dulk M, Meerchoek-Klein E, et al. Improved survival after resectable non-cardia gastric cancer in the Netherlands: the importance of surgical training and quality control. Eur J Surg Oncol 2009;35(7):718; with permission)

FUTURE DIRECTION OF GASTRIC CANCER SURGERY

Considering the declining incidence of gastric cancer and the learning curve for the procedure, it is not logical to educate and maintain all surgeons in the D2 nodal gastrectomy procedure in Western countries. For operative quality assurance, training dedicated surgeons for adequate performance of the procedure and regionalizing the care of this difficult disease may improve overall quality of care and, potentially, overall survival.

REFERENCES

1. Japanese Gastric Cancer Association. Guidelines for diagnosis and treatment of carcinoma of the stomach. Japanese Gastric Cancer Association; 2004. Available at: http://www.jgca.jp/PDFfiles/Guidelines2004_eng.pdf. Accessed June 14, 2011.
2. Songun I, Putter H, Kranenbarg EM, et al. Surgical treatment of gastric cancer: 15-year follow-up results of the randomized nationwide Dutch D1D2 trial. Lancet Oncol 2010;11(5):439–49.
3. Edge SB, Byrd DR, Compton CC, et al. American Joint Committee on Cancer. Stomach. In: AJCC cancer staging manual. 7th edition. New York: Springer; 2010. p. 117–26.
4. Japanese Gastric Cancer Association. Japanese gastric cancer treatment guidelines 2010 (ver.3). Gastric Cancer 2011;14:113–23.
5. Japanese Gastric Cancer Association. Japanese Classification of Gastric Carcinoma: 3rd English edition. Gastric Cancer 2011;14:101–12.
6. Yamaguchi S, Kuroyanagi H, Milson JW, et al. Venous anatomy of the right colon. precise structure of the major vein and gastrocolic trunk in 58 cadavers. Dis Colon Rectum 2001;45:1337–40.
7. Kawasaki K, Kanaji S, Kobayashi I, et al. Multidetector computed tomography for preoperative identification of left gastric vein location in patients with gastric cancer. Gastric Cancer 2010;13:25–9.
8. Natsume T, Shuto K, Yanagawa N, et al. The classification of anatomic variations in the perigastric vessels by dual-phase CT to reduce intraoperative bleeding during laparoscopic gastrectomy. Surg Endosc 2011;25(5):1420–4.
9. Okabayashi T, Kobayashi M, Nishimori I, et al. Autopsy study of anatomical features of the posterior gastric artery for surgical contribution. World J Gastroenterol 2006;12(33):5357–9.
10. Loukas M, Wartmann CT, Louis RG Jr, et al. The clinical anatomy of the posterior gastric artery revisited. Surg Radiol Anat 2007;29:361–6.
11. Sano T, Yamamoto S, Sasako M. Randomized controlled trial to evaluate spelenectomy in total gastrectomy for proximal gastric carcinoma: Japan Clinical Oncology Group study JCOG 0110-MF. Jpn J Clin Oncol 2002;32(9):363–4.
12. Hundahl SA, Macdonald JS, Benedetti J, et al. Surgical treatment variation in a prospective, randomized trial of chemoradiotherapy in gastric cancer: the effect of undertreatment. Ann Surg Oncol 2002;9(3):278–86.
13. Bollschweiler E, Boettcher K, Hoelscher AH, et al. Preoperative assessment of lymph node metastases in patients with gastric cancer: evaluation of the Maruyama computer program. Br J Surg 1992;79(2):156–60.
14. Peeters KC, Hundahl SA, Kranenbarg EK, et al. Low Maruyama Index surgery for gastric cancer: blinded reanalysis of the Dutch D1-D2 trial. World J Surg 2005;29(12):1576–84.
15. Hundahl SA, Peeters KC, Kranenbarg EK, et al. Improved regional control and survival with "low Maruyama Index" surgery in gastric cancer: autopsy findings from the Dutch D1-D2 Trial. Gastric Cancer 2007;10(2):84–6.

16. Kong SH, Yoo MW, Kim JW, et al. Validation of limited lymphadenectomy for lower-third gastric cancer based on depth of tumour invasion. Br J Surg 2011; 98(1):65–72.
17. Cuschieri A, Weeden S, Fielding J, et al. Patient survival after D1 and D2 resections for gastric cancer: long-term results of the MRC randomized surgical trial. Br J Cancer 1999;79(9–10):1522–30.
18. Bonenkamp JJ, Hermans J, Sasako M, et al. Extended lymph-node dissection for gastric cancer. N Engl J Med 1999;340:908–14.
19. Bonenkamp JJ, Hermans J, Sasako M, et al. Quality control of lymph node dissection in the Dutch randomized trial of D1 and D2 lymph node dissection for gastric cancer. Gastric Cancer 1998;1:152–9.
20. Lee JH, Ryu KW, Lee J, et al. Learning curve for total gastrectomy with D2 lymph node dissection: cumulative sum analysis for qualified surgery. Ann Surg Oncol 2006;13(9):1175–81.
21. Parikh D, Johnson M, Chagla L, et al. D2 gastrectomy: lessons from a prospective audit of the learning curve. Br J Surg 1996;83:1595–9.
22. Tsujinaka T, Sasako M, Yamamoto S, et al. Influence of overweight on surgical complications for gastric cancer: results from a randomized control trial comparing D2 and extended para-aortic D3 lymphadenectomy (JCOG9501). Ann Surg Oncol 2007;14(2):355–61.
23. Krijnen P, den Dulk M, Meerchoek-Klein E, et al. Improved survival after resectable non-cardia gastric cancer in the Netherlands: the importance of surgical training and quality control. Eur J Surg Oncol 2009;35(7):715–20.

Gastric Cancer Eastern Experience

Mitsuru Sasako, MD

KEYWORDS

• Gastric cancer surgery • D2 dissection • Stage migration
• Quality of lymphadenectomy • Quality of postoperative care
• Splenectomy

GUIDELINES FOR THE STANDARD TREATMENT OF GASTRIC CANCER

Several guidelines are used for cancer therapy throughout the world. In the Japan Gastric Cancer Association (JGCA) guideline, standard surgery for T2 to T4 curable gastric cancer is defined as more than two-thirds gastrectomy with D2 dissection.[1] In the 2010 European Society of Medical Oncology's guideline, the standard surgery for curable gastric cancer is the D2 gastrectomy.[2] Of note, this is the first time this society has clearly advocated for the D2 approach. The National Comprehensive Cancer Network (NCCN) guidelines, commonly followed in the United States, recommend that gastric resections include regional lymphadenectomy to include the perigastric lymph nodes (D1) and those along the named vessels of the celiac axis (D2), with a goal of examining at least 15 or more lymph nodes.[3]

STAGE-SPECIFIC RESULTS OF RESECTED GASTRIC CANCER IN THE WEST AND EAST

The JGCA-maintained registry analyzed a total of 11,261 patients who underwent gastric resection in 2001.[4] The 5-year overall survival (OS) by UICC TNM stage (sixth version) was as follows: stage IA, 91.8%; stage IB, 84.6%; stage II, 70.5%; stage IIIA, 46.6%; stage IIIB, 29.9%; stage IV, 16.6%. Although the standard treatment at that time was surgery alone[5], an unknown proportion of those undergoing surgery may also have received adjuvant treatment either through enrollment into clinical trials or by doctor's or patient's choice.

Another available source of information regarding gastric cancer survival is obtained through single-institution reporting. Five-year OS after a total gastrectomy of 881 patients undergoing a total gastrectomy between 1995 and 2001 at Asan Medical Center, Korea, was 94.6%, 90.8%, 76.7%, 55.7%, 41.3%, and 15.4% for stage IA, IB, II, IIIA, IIIB, and IV, respectively.[6] From another Korean institution, National Seoul University Hospital, the results of 10,783 consecutive patients who were surgically treated

COI: The author has nothing to disclose in connection with this article.
Department of Surgery, Hyogo College of Medicine, 1-1, Mukogawacho, Nishinomiya, Hyogo 663-8501, Japan
E-mail address: msasako@hyo-med.ac.jp

Surg Oncol Clin N Am 21 (2012) 71–77
doi:10.1016/j.soc.2011.09.013
1055-3207/12/$ – see front matter © 2012 Elsevier Inc. All rights reserved.

surgonc.theclinics.com

between 1970 and 1996 were reported. Five-year OS was 92.9%, 84.2%, 69.3%, 45.8%, 29.6%, and 9.2% for stage IA, IB, II, IIIA, IIIB, and IV, respectively.[7] Differences in these results seem attributable mainly to the period of inclusion and improvement over time. Selection bias hampers straight comparison with nationwide registry.

The nationwide results of the United States by the National Cancer Data Base (NCDB) were reported for the cohort treated between 1985 and 1996.[8] Stage-specific OS was 78%, 58%, 34%, 20%, 8%, and 7% for stage IA, IB, II, IIIA, IIIB, and IV, respectively (**Table 1**). More recent data, after the results of Intergroup study 0116 (INT 0116), have yet to be published in medical journals. According to the report by Enestvedt and colleagues,[9] 36.8% of patients surgically staged from IB to III under-went adjuvant chemoradiotherapy after gastric resection between 2001 and 2006 in the state of Oregon. Stage-specific 5-year OS was approximately 13%, 13%, and 5% for stage IB, II, and III, respectively. These results are unacceptably poor, explained by the extremely low percentage of proper adjuvant treatment, correct staging, or adequate surgery. With this kind of data base it is not easy to obtain the precise details of patients' background, and comparison is not easy.

OVERALL SURVIVAL IN VARIOUS CLINICAL TRIALS IN THE WEST AND EAST

To know exactly the stage-specific OS by surgery alone, the most reliable way is to analyze the results of the surgery-alone arm of clinical trials that have evaluated some kind of new treatment in comparison with a surgery-alone arm as control. Since 2007, when the results of INT-0116,[10] the MAGIC trial,[11] and ACTS-GC[12] became available, it has become difficult to carry out a randomized controlled trial (RCT) having surgery alone as control.

In Japan the results of the surgery-alone arm of the ACTS-GC study, in which 1059 patients were enrolled, are available. In this trial, only stage II and IIIA/B by the Japanese classification were included. These patients can be restaged by UICC TNM classification. Some patients in stage III in the Japanese classification were clas-sified as stage IV by TNM classification. Five-year OS was 70.8%, 56.2%, 40.1%, and 42.7% for UICC stage II, IIIA, IIIB, and IV, respectively in the surgery-only group.[13] In the Dutch Gastric Cancer Study, the 5-year OS was 81%, 61%, 42%, 28%, 13%, and 28%, for stage IA, IB, II, IIIA, IIIB, and IV, respectively.[14] Although the Italian Gastric Cancer Study was a phase 2 study, they reported stage-specific survival due to a larger number of patients included.[15] As shown in **Table 2**, their results are some-where between those of the ACTS-GC and the Dutch study.

Table 1
Stage-specific 5-year overall survival rate (%) of cancer registries and a large case series

	JGCA Registry	SNUH	NCDB
Period	2001	1970–1996	1985–1996
Stage IA	91.8	92.9	78
Stage IB	84.6	84.2	58
Stage II	70.5	69.3	34
Stage IIIA	46.6	45.8	20
Stage IIIB	29.9	29.6	8
Stage IV	16.6	9.2	7
Total patients	11261	10783	49756

Abbreviations: JGCA, Japan Gastric Cancer Association; NCDB, National Cancer Data Base; SNUH, Seoul National University Hospital.

Table 2
Stage-specific 5-year overall survival rate (%) of D2 surgery in clinical trials

	ACTS-GC[13]	Dutch D1 vs D2[14]	Italian P2[15]
Stage IA		81 (69)	95.0 (53)
Stage IB		61 (64)	87.5 (22)
Stage II	70.2 (278)	42 (66)	57.5 (31)
Stage IIIA	56.2 (153)	28 (72)	42.5 (37)
Stage IIIB	40.1 (53)	13 (39)	22.5 (25)
Stage IV	42.7 (35)	28 (18)	2.5 (23)
Total patients	519	328	191

Numbers in parentheses show number of patients for each stage.
Abbreviation: ACTS-GC, Adjuvant Chemotherapy Trial of TS-1 for Gastric Cancer.

In other clinical trials,[16–19] stage-specific OS cannot be obtained in publications but they would not be reliable, if available, because of the small numbers in each stage in these trials as compared with the ACTS-GC. Careful comparison of the patients' background may suggest some difference in these results. **Table 3** shows the background of the patients enrolled in the surgery-alone arm of these studies. Compared with the results of Western trials, much better OS are shown in Japanese trials (see **Table 3**).

STAGE MIGRATION: FACT AND SOURCE OF MIGRATION

Stage migration is a hampering factor when trying to compare the stage-specific results of different countries where the accuracy of staging is different. Wider lymph node dissection and more accurate lymph retrieval from the specimen result in more accurate staging, which in turn results in better stage-specific survival. Bunt and colleagues[20] evaluated the effect of stage migration in the Dutch study where D1 and D2 dissection were compared. If the patients who underwent D2 dissection were restaged abandoning the information about N2 level, 72 of 214 (34%) would have a different stage due to stage migration. Using the reported Japanese stage-specific survival results, calculated stage-specific survival by D2 staging is better in each stage than that of calculated stage-specific survival if N2 information is not used for staging. Especially in stage IIIA and IIIB, as much as 15% difference could be expected between these two staging systems. In the Japan Clinical Oncology Group (JCOG) study 9501 where D2 and D2+ para-aortic node dissection were compared, similar stage migration was observed. However, the incidence of para-aortic node metastasis (8.8%) is much smaller than that of N2 nodes, therefore only 8.5% of the entire patient cohort who underwent D3 dissection could have been restaged by abandoning the N3 information.[21]

In the Dutch study it was found that not only the extent of nodal dissection but also the way of retrieving nodes and the effort of pathologists resulted in stage migration.[22] Similarly, how the resected stomach is examined may be a source of stage migration. If the deepest part of the region is not histologically examined, earlier T stage would be attributed to these lesions.

SPLENECTOMY

In both the Dutch and the Medical Research Council (MRC) study comparing D1 with D2 surgery, splenectomy was found to be more relevant than D2 itself, due to higher

Table 3
Comparison of patients' characteristics, background, treatment, and 5-year overall survival in the surgery-alone arm of clinical trials

	JCOG 9206-2[16]	JCOG 9501[17]	INT-0116[10]	MAGIC[11]	EORCT 40954[18]	FNCLCC/FFCD[19]
No. of patients	133	523	275	253 (204)	72 (68)	110 (98)
Tumor location (%)						
L/M/U/W	39/44/37/12	217/206/100/0	154/69/50/0	NA	15/18/39	NA
Histological type (%)						
Dif/undif	43/88	204/316	77/128/70	NA	39/33	NA
pT stage (1/2/3/4)	2/39/88/4	23/257/230/13	22/63/168/22	16/55/106/16	4/30/24/7	27//58[a]
% pT3/4	69%	46%	65%	63%	48%	68%
pN (±)	101/32	348/175	231/44	114/42	52/13	68/17
% Node positive	76%	67%	84%	73%	80%	80%
Median size	5.5	5.5	NA	5.0	NA	NA
Surgery <D2/≧D2 (%)	0/132	0/523	254/20	70/96	5/63	NA
R0 resection	100%	100%	100%?	66%	67%	74%
5-Year OS	61%	70%	~25%	23%	~50%	24%

Abbreviations: Dif, differentiated; L/M/U/W, Distal part/Middle part/Proximal part/Whole stomach; NA, not available; OS, overall survival; undif, undifferentiated.
[a] T1 + 2//T3 + 4: numbers of T1 and T2 versus T3 and T4.

postoperative mortality.[23,24] In these trials, the protocol required the surgeons to carry out a splenopancreatectomy in case of a total gastrectomy in the D2 arm. Therefore, the majority of those who underwent total gastrectomy received splenectomy and distal pancreatectomy. Because of misunderstanding of the Japanese classification and definition of D category, even some patients who underwent a distal gastrectomy received splenectomy in these trials, which resulted in high mortality due to remnant stomach necrosis.[23]

Moreover, the worse prognosis of the D2 group was attributed to splenectomy in MRC trials comparing two groups of patients who underwent splenectomy or not.[25] However, it is known that prognosis of tumors located in the upper part of the stomach is worse than that of distally located tumors. The larger the tumor, the more frequently they require a total gastrectomy. These factors, biology of proximal tumor and size of tumors, seem to strongly affect the survival results. To avoid such bias, only an RCT comparing a total gastrectomy with and without splenectomy can provide a proper conclusion to this question. The JCOG performed an RCT to evaluate the noninferiority of spleen-preserving total gastrectomy to a pancreas-preserving total gastrectomy with splenectomy for patients who had T2 or deeper tumors in the proximal part of the stomach, requiring a total gastrectomy.[26] Sano and colleagues[27] reported more blood loss and higher morbidity after splenectomy, but no difference in mortality in experienced surgeons' hands. Long-term results are awaited.

IMPACT OF D2 DISSECTION ON THE RESULTS OF ADJUVANT TREATMENT

In the INT-0116 study, subgroup analysis by extent of lymphadenectomy revealed that the effect of adjuvant chemoradiation depends on the type of lymphadenectomy. Due to the limited number of those undergoing D2 dissection in this study, interaction between treatment effect and type of lymphadenectomy was not statistically significant, but those with D2 dissection did not show any benefit of adjuvant chemoradiation. These results were later transformed into the correlation between Maruyama Index (a computer program–based probability calculation of nodal residual disease) and the survival results of the patients in this study.[28] Dikken and colleagues[29] reported the influence of the extent of lymphadenectomy on the pattern of recurrence and OS in comparison with chemoradiotherapy. The investigators suggested that effect of chemoradiotherapy depends on type of lymphadenectomy, and that postoperative adjuvant chemoradiotherapy might compensate nonradical surgery for better local control.

Historically only two pivotal studies were able to show the benefit of adjuvant chemotherapy, the ACTS-GC study[12] and the CLASSIC study.[30] In these studies, all patients underwent D2 dissection as local control. The effect of radiotherapy added to adjuvant chemotherapy is being tested in two clinical trials.[31] The CRITICS trial is a European study launched in the Netherlands, wherein the effect of postoperative chemoradiotherapy (capecitabine + cisplatin with 45 Gy radiation) is compared with postoperative chemotherapy alone in the course of European standard perioperative treatment (preoperative chemotherapy comprising 3 courses of epirubicin + cisplatin + capecitabine and D1+ surgery followed by postoperative chemotherapy [same as the preoperative one]). This study is still open for accrual.[31] Another study is the ARTIST trial, a Korean single-institutional study, which compares postoperative adjuvant therapy by capecitabine + cisplatin with or without simultaneous radiotherapy. All patients should undergo D2 dissection. Four hundred and fifty-eight patients were enrolled between October 2004 and April 2008, and the short-term results, mainly concerning the safety profile, were reported in ASCO-GI 2009.[32] The final results are yet to be reported.

SUMMARY

In the East, D2 dissection shows much better results than less extended surgery followed by adjuvant treatment. Adjuvant chemotherapy without radiotherapy show significantly better survival results than surgery alone only when D2 dissection is applied. Without good local control, including regional lymph node metastasis, cure rate cannot be high.

REFERENCES

1. Japanese Gastric Cancer Association. Japanese gastric cancer treatment guidelines 2010 (ver.3). Gastric Cancer 2011;14:113–23.
2. Okines A, Verheij M, Allum W, et al. Gastric cancer: ESMO clinical practice guideline for diagnosis, treatment and follow-up. Ann Oncol 2010;21(Suppl 5):v50–4.
3. Version 2. Available at: http://www.nccn.org/professionals/physician_gls/pdf/gastric.pdf. Accessed October 19, 2011.
4. Isobe Y, Nashimoto A, Akazawa K, et al. Gastric cancer treatment in Japan: 2008 annual report of the JGCA nationwide registry. Gastric Cancer. DOI:10.1007/s10120-011-0085-6. [Epub ahead of print].
5. Sasako M. The gastric cancer treatment guideline. In: Kaminishi M, Takubo K, Mafune K, editors. The diversity of gastric cancer. Tokyo: Springer; 2005. p. 235–41.
6. Cheong O, Kim BS, Yook JH, et al. Modified radical lymphadenectomy without splenectomy in patients with proximal gastric cancer: comparison with standard D2 lymphadenectomy for distal gastric cancer. J Surg Oncol 2008;98:500–4.
7. Kim JP, Lee JH, Kim SJ, et al. Clinicopathologic characteristics and prognostic factors in 10783 patients with gastric cancer. Gastric Cancer 1998;1:125–33.
8. Hundahl S, Phillips JL, Menck HR. The National Cancer Data Base report on poor survival of U.S. gastric carcinoma patients treated with gastrectomy. Cancer 2000;88:921–32.
9. Enestvedt CK, Diggs BS, Shipley DK, et al. A population-based analysis of surgical and adjuvant therapy for resected gastric cancer: are patients receiving appropriate treatment following publication of the Intergroup 0116 results? Gastrointest Cancer Res 2009;3:233–8.
10. Macdonald JS, Smalley SR, Benedetti J, et al. Chemoradiotherapy after surgery compared with surgery alone for adenocarcinoma of the stomach and gastroesophageal junction. N Engl J Med 2001;345:725–30.
11. Cunningham D, Allum WH, Stenning SP, et al. Perioperative chemotherapy versus surgery alone for resectable gastroesophageal cancer. N Engl J Med 2006;355:11–20.
12. Sakuramoto S, Sasako M, Yamaguchi T, et al. Adjuvant chemotherapy for gastric cancer with S-1, an oral fluoropyrimidine. N Engl J Med 2007;357:1810–20.
13. Sasako M, Sakuramoto S, Katai H, et al. Five-year outcomes of randomized phase III trial comparing adjuvant chemotherapy with S-1 versus surgery alone in stage II/III gastric cancer; ACTS-GC. J Clin Oncol 2011. DOI:10.1200/JCO.2011.36.5908. [Epub ahead of print].
14. Bonenkamp JJ, Hermans J, Sasako M, et al. Extended lymph-node dissection for gastric cancer. N Engl J Med 1999;340:908–14.
15. Degiuli M, Sasako M, Ponti A, et al. Survival results of a multicentre phase II study to evaluate D2 gastrectomy for gastric cancer. Br J Cancer 2004;90:1727–32.
16. Miyashiro I, Furukawa H, Sasako M, et al. Randomized clinical trial of adjuvant chemotherapy with intraperitoneal and intravenous cisplatin followed by oral fluorouracil (UFT) in serosa-positive gastric cancer versus curative resection

alone: final results of Japan Clinical Oncology Group trial JCOG9206-2. Gastric Cancer 2011;14(3):212–8.

17. Sasako M, Sano T, Yamamoto S, et al. D2 lymphadenectomy alone or with para-aortic nodal dissection for gastric cancer. N Engl J Med 2008;359:453–62.

18. Schumacher C, Gretschel S, Lordick F, et al. Neoadjuvant chemotherapy compared with surgery alone for locally advanced cancer of the stomach and cardia: European Organization for Research and Treatment of Cancer randomized trial 40954. J Clin Oncol 2010;28:5210–8.

19. Ychou M, Boige V, Pignon JP, et al. Perioperative chemotherapy compared with surgery alone for resectable gastroesophageal adenocarcinoma: an FNCLCC and FFCD multicenter phase III trial. J Clin Oncol 2011;29:1715–21.

20. Bunt AM, Hermans J, Smit VT, et al. Surgical/pathological stage migration confounds comparisons of gastric cancer survival rates between Japan and Western countries. J Clin Oncol 1995;13:19–25.

21. Yoshikawa T, Sasako M, Sano T, et al. Stage migration caused by D2 dissection with para-aortic lymphadenectomy for gastric cancer from the results of a prospective randomized controlled trial. Br J Surg 2006;93:1526–9.

22. Bunt AM, Hermans J, van de Velde CJ, et al. Lymph node retrieval in a randomized trial on Western-type versus Japanese-type surgery in gastric cancer. J Clin Oncol 1996;14:2289–94.

23. Sasako M. Risk factors for surgical treatment in the Dutch gastric cancer trial. Br J Surg 1997;84:1567–71.

24. Cuscheiri A, Fayers P, Craven J, et al. Postoperative morbidity and mortality after D1 and D2 resections for gastric cancer: preliminary results of the MRC randomised controlled surgical trial. Lancet 1996;347:995–9.

25. Cuschieri A, Weeden S, Fielding J, et al. Patient survival after D1 and D2 resection for gastric cancer: long-term results of the MRC randomised surgical trial. Br J Cancer 1999;79:1522–30.

26. Sano T, Yamamoto S, Sasako M. Randomized controlled trial to evaluate splenectomy in total gastrectomy for proximal gastric carcinoma: Japan Clinical Oncology Group Study JCOG 0110-MF. Jpn J Clin Oncol 2002;32:363–4.

27. Sano T, Sasako M, Shibata T, et al. Randomized controlled trial to evaluate splenectomy in total gastrectomy for proximal gastric carcinoma (JCOG0110): analyses of operative morbidity, operation time, and blood loss. J Clin Oncol 2010; 28(15s):305s.

28. Hundahl SA, Macdonald JS, Benedetti J, et al. Surgical treatment variation in a prospective, randomized trial of chemoradiotherapy in gastric cancer: the effect of undertreatment. Ann Surg Oncol 2002;9:278–86.

29. Dikken JL, Jansen EP, Cats A, et al. Impact of the extent of surgery and postoperative chemoradiotherapy on recurrence patterns in gastric cancer. J Clin Oncol 2010;28:2430–6.

30. Bang Y. Adjuvant capecitabine and oxaliplatin for gastric cancer: results of the phase III CLASSIC trial. J Clin Oncol 2011;29(18s):780s.

31. Den Dulk M, Verheij M, Cats A, et al. The essentials of locoregional control in the treatment of gastric cancer. Scand J Surg 2006;95:236–42.

32. Lee J, Kang W, Lim D, et al. Phase III trial of adjuvant capecitabine/cisplatin (XP) compared with capecitabine/cisplatin/RT (XPRT) in resected gastric cancer with D2 nodal dissection (ARTIST trial): safety analysis. Abstract, 2011 gastrointestinal Cancer Symposium (ASCO-GI). Richmond: Cadmus Professional Communications, a Cenveo Company.

Surgery for Gastric Cancer: What the Trials Indicate

Scott A. Hundahl, MD

KEYWORDS

- Gastric cancer • Surgery • Trials • Lymphadenectomy

To optimize the therapeutic value of an operation for cancer, surgeons must weigh survival value on one hand against mortality/morbidity risk on the other. As a result of several prospective, randomized trials, many surgeons view the muddied waters of international opinion concerning optimal gastric cancer treatment as having been filtered clean. But does this view withstand detailed scrutiny? Unquestionably, the reflexively-radical surgical hubris of yore has given way to a more nuanced, customized approach to this disease. Emphasizing existing trial findings and controversies, this review hopes to illuminate the topic so the reader can reach his own conclusions.

EAST-WEST DIFFERENCES IN DIAGNOSIS AND STAGING

East-West differences in gastric cancer have been commented on but it is not always realized that even the histologic diagnosis of gastric cancer varies. For example, noninvasive mucosal disease is routinely categorized as early gastric cancer according to the Japanese General Rules for Gastric Cancer Study, but as simple dysplasia or carcinoma in situ by Western pathologists. Western pathologists are reluctant to diagnose gastric cancer unless they identify microscopic invasion of the basement membrane lamina propria. The so-called Vienna Classification explicitly documents and addresses these major diagnostic differences.[1] The new Group Classification incorporated into the Japanese Classification of Gastric Carcinoma (see later discussion) classifies lesions into 5 categories, from benign to obviously neoplastic, and this should remedy the problem.[2]

Complications such as obstruction, bleeding, or perforation only infrequently prompt an emergency operation for gastric cancer. In the modern era, clinical staging drives treatment and such treatment is customized. Extent-of-disease evaluation for gastric cancer generally includes upper endoscopy with biopsy, endoscopic ultrasound, spiral computed tomography (CT) of the abdomen/pelvis, and a chest radiograph or chest CT. Laparoscopy has a role in the staging and treatment of selected

Department of Surgery, U.C. Davis, VA Northern California Health Care System, Sacramento VA at Mather 10535, Hospital Way (112), Mather, CA 95655-1200, USA
E-mail addresses: shundahl@comcast.net; scott.hundahl@va.gov

Surg Oncol Clin N Am 21 (2012) 79–97
doi:10.1016/j.soc.2011.09.005
1055-3207/12/$ – see front matter Published by Elsevier Inc.
surgonc.theclinics.com

cases, particularly in ruling out peritoneal dissemination or extraregional disease. Positron emission tomography (PET) scanning for gastric cancer (as opposed to esophageal cancer or gastroesophageal junction cancer) is controversial. The performance characteristics of fluorodeoxyglucose (FDG)-PET scanning for gastric cancer are not as good as for other neoplasms.[3] For example, only 60% to 75% of primary gastric tumors have a suspicious standardized uptake value.[4,5]

The current seventh edition of American Joint Commission for Cancer (AJCC)/Union for International Cancer Control (UICC) staging, to be used for all cases after January 1, 2010, represents a major departure from previous versions. For example, tumors arising from the proximal 5 cm of the stomach but extending to the gastroesophageal junction, as well as all esophagogastric junction tumors, are now classified for staging purposes as esophageal cancer (ie, not stomach).[6,7] Combined with other changes, this has created substantial migration of both site and stage, compared with previous editions. Unintended consequences relating to treatment have appeared. These consequences will likely be addressed in future AJCC/UICC editions. For the purpose of this article, gastric adenocarcinoma is staged/classified according to modern seventh edition mandates.

A second staging issue should be highlighted. The Japanese Gastric Cancer Association (JGCA) staging (also termed the Updated General Rules, based on the title of the first English version published in 1981[8]) represents an internationally popular alternative staging system used throughout Asia and many other areas of the world. This popular system, with its previously anatomic classification of lymph nodes, was initially designed not only to assess prognosis but to guide surgical treatment. This system has undergone extensive revision over the years as the recommended surgical treatment of regional lymph nodes has changed.[9] It was not until 2001 that treatment guidelines began to be disconnected from the staging system.[10,11] In 1997, with the publication of the 13th edition of the JGCA Staging Guidelines, the N4 (para-aortic) designation was eliminated, and, with it, the term D4 lymphadenectomy. With the change, the earlier N4 para-aortic disease became the newly defined N3 level. In the most recent 2011 version, the N3 category has also been eliminated.[2,11] Given the redefinition of N2 nodes, a pre-1997 D3 lymphadenectomy is now a D2 lymphadenectomy. The modern D2 lymphadenectomy addresses regional node stations 1 to 12; nodal disease outside these node stations is now classified as metastatic M1 disease.[2] To clarify the current definitions, the JGCA published an updated third English version in 2011,[2,11] accompanied by separate algorithmic treatment guidelines,[11] which should remedy the currently widespread international confusion.[10] An additional advantage of this 2011 version is that final staging is now, for the first time, based on numbers of nodes involved and is in agreement with AJCC/UICC tumor- node, metastasis (TNM) staging definitions.[6,7]

Modern JGCA D-level lymphadenectomy definitions are driven by whether a (mandated) total gastrectomy or distal gastrectomy is performed, based on primary tumor characteristics. For total gastrectomy, a D2 lymphadenectomy is now defined as complete removal of node stations 1 to 7, 8a, 9 to 11, and 12a. For DISTAL gastrectomy, D2 lymphadenectomy is now defined as complete removal of node stations 1, 3, 4sb and 4d, 5 to 7, 8a, 9, 11p, and 12a (**Fig. 1**).[11]

EXTENT OF ORGAN RESECTION. PROSPECTIVE RANDOMIZED TRAILS ADDRESSING ROUTINE TOTAL GASTRECTOMY VERSUS SUBTOTAL GASTRECTOMY

The French Subtotal versus Total Gastrectomy Trial, by Gouzi and colleagues[12] for the French Association for Surgical Research, was conducted between 1980 and 1985 to

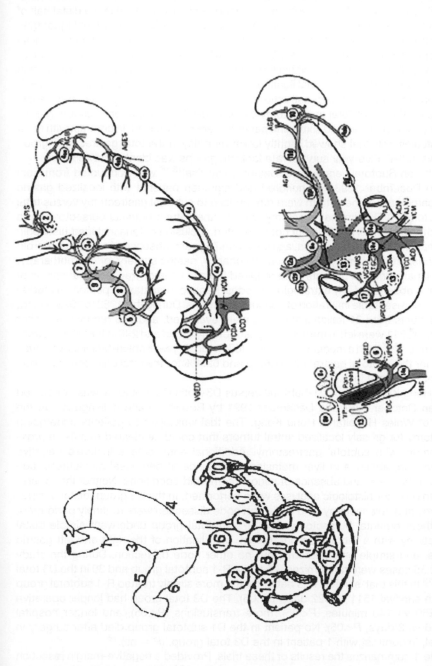

Fig. 1. JGCA-defined lymph node stations, according to the 2011 Japanese Classification of Gastric Carcinoma: 3rd English Edition.[2] For total gastrectomy, a D2 lymphadenectomy is now defined as complete removal of node stations 1 to 7, 8a, 9 to 11, and 12a. For distal gastrectomy, a D2 lymphadenectomy is now defined as complete removal of node stations 1, 3, 4sb and 4d, 5 to 7, 8a, 9, 11p, and 12a. (*From* Japanese Gastric Cancer Association. Japanese gastric cancer treatment guidelines 2010 (ver. 3). Gastric Cancer 2011;14(2):113–23; with permission.)

address the potential value of routine total gastrectomy versus the higher mortality and morbidity associated with this procedure, as documented by McNeer[13,14] and others. Eligibility criteria included presence of an adenocarcinoma located in the distal half of the stomach, good organ function, and no evidence of nodal involvement higher than the gastroesophageal junction or in the splenopancreatic region. Cases of superficial carcinoma (in situ or early T1) were to be excluded, as were cases of obvious linitis plastica–type extensive infiltration within the gastric wall. Extensive lymph node dissection was not mandated, but proximal ligation/resection of the left gastric artery was. A Billroth II gastrojejunostomy reconstruction was used for all subtotal gastrectomy cases. Reconstruction for all total gastrectomy cases consisted of Roux-en-Y esophagojejunostomy. One-hundred and sixty-nine patients were randomized. In contrast with most other studies, this trial showed slightly lower mortality in the total gastrectomy group (1.3% vs 3.2%). Five-year survival rate for both groups was identical at 48%.[12]

The Italian Subtotal versus Total Gastrectomy Trial[15,16] was conducted from April 1982 to December 1993. Six-hundred and eighteen patients with localized gastric adenocarcinoma of the antrum were randomized to subtotal gastrectomy versus total gastrectomy. A D2 lymphadenectomy and Japanese-type omental bursectomy was recommended for all patients but not mandated. Inclusion criteria included histologic confirmation of adenocarcinoma, age less than 75 years, absence of serious comorbid conditions, and no history of previous malignancy, gastric surgery, or chemotherapy. During laparotomy, all patients were required to have a tumor-free proximal margin of 6 cm, and absence of any extraregional nodes, hepatic metastases, peritoneal metastases, or unresectable infiltration of contiguous organs. During this 1982 to 1993 period, 1372 patients from 31 Italian institutions were evaluated, and 648 randomized; after exclusions, 311 were left in the subtotal gastrectomy group and 296 in the total gastrectomy group.[16,17] With a median 72 months' follow-up, 5-year Kaplan-Meier survival was 65.3% for the subtotal gastrectomy group and 62.4% for the total gastrectomy group (P = not significant [ns]).[16,17]

The Hong Kong Trial of D1-Subtotal versus D3-Total Gastrectomy was conducted between October 1987 and December 1991 by Robertson and colleagues[18] at the Prince of Wales Hospital in Hong Kong. The trial was open to patients undergoing laparotomy for grossly localized antral tumors that could be cleared to a 6-cm proximal margin with subtotal gastrectomy. Additional entry criteria included negative distal margin, absence of liver metastases, absence of peritoneal metastases, age less than 75 years, and absence of serious comorbid conditions. Neither intraoperative cytologic nor histologic analyses were performed. In the D3 group, distal pancreatectomy and splenectomy, and D3 lymph node dissection were routinely performed, but without omental bursectomy. The R-1-subtotal group underwent simple distal gastrectomy with a 6-cm proximal margin, high ligation of the right and left gastric arteries, and simple omentectomy, but no other node dissection. During the study period, 55 cases were randomized, 25 in the R-1 subtotal group and 30 in the D3 total group.[18] In this trial, survival was better for the more simply treated R-1 subtotal group (median survival 1511 vs 922 days, $P<.05$). The D3 total group had longer operative time (260 vs 140 minutes, $P<.05$), more transfusions ($P<.05$), and longer hospital stay (16 vs 8 days, $P<.05$). No patient in the D1 subtotal group died after surgery in hospital, in contrast with 1 patient in the D3 total group. (P = ns).[18]

Table 1 summarizes the results of these trials. Provided a negative-margin resection can be obtained with a subtotal gastrectomy, and provided it is not a linitis plastica situation (ie, diffuse infiltrating poorly differentiated cancer eliciting a leather-bottle stomach), routine total gastrectomy is to be avoided. The 2010 Japanese treatment guidelines, and the 2011 English version, call for a proximal margin of 3 cm from gross disease for

Table 1
Prospective randomized clinical trials: total versus subtotal gastrectomy

Total vs Subtotal Trials		Inclusion Criteria	Mortality/ Survival	Mortality/ Survival	P Value (Survival)
			Subtotal	Total	
Gouzi et al[12]	N = 169	Antral tumor M-0	3%/48% (5-y survival)	1%/48% (5-y survival)	ns
Bozzetti et al[15]	N = 618	>6 cm proximal margin possible M-0	1%/65% (5-y survival)	2%/62% (5-y survival)	ns
			Subtotal+D1	Total+D = 3	
Robertson et al[18]	N = 55	Antral >6 cm margin M-0, age <75 y	0%/1511 d median survival	3%/922 d median survival	0.04 0.07

Abbreviation: ns, not significant.

localized well-circumscribed Borrmann I or II tumors, and a margin of at least 5 cm for other tumors.[11] Total gastrectomy is performed whenever necessary to meet these requirements. Total gastrectomy should also be performed for cases of linitis plastica.

IN SITU AND T-1 DISEASE: ROLE OF ENDOSCOPIC MUCOSAL/SUBMUCOSAL RESECTION

For a selected superficial early gastric cancer (ie, Tis or T-1 tumor), endoscopic mucosal resection (EMR) has emerged as a reasonable option.[19–24] In the classic technique of EMR, a submucosal injection of saline floats the area of tumor-bearing mucosa off the underlying muscularis propria and the lesion is resected with a special cautery snare with hooks to preserve specimen orientation for margin analysis. The procedure can be technically challenging, but innovations such as use of incision endoforceps,[25] aspiration mucosectomy,[26] use of a stabilizing distal magnetic anchor,[27,28] and use of double endoscope resection techniques[29] can facilitate it. In endoscopic submucosal resection (ESR), the margins of resection are first circum-scribed using a high-frequency electric knife and the submucosal layer specifically dissected from the muscularis propria layer.[11]

Selection of cases suitable for EMR/ESR depends on the absence of disease in the regional lymphatics. A article paper by Gotoda and colleagues[30] concerning 5265 surgically treated T-1 cases from the National Cancer Center Hospital and the Cancer Institute Hospital in Tokyo offers guidance. For intramucosal tumors, none of 1230 well-differentiated cancers of less than 30-mm diameter, regardless of ulceration find-ings, were associated with nodal involvement. Regardless of tumor size, for completely intramucosal tumors, none of 929 cancers without ulceration were associ-ated with nodal metastases. For submucosal cancers, there was a significant correla-tion between tumor size larger than 30 mm and lymphatic-vascular involvement, with an increased risk of nodal involvement. However, none of the 145 well-differentiated adenocarcinomas of less than 30-mm diameter without lymphatic or venous perme-ation were associated with nodal involvement, provided that the lesion had invaded less than 500 μm into the submucosa.[30]

In an 11-year, 445-case series by Ono and colleagues[19] from the National Cancer Center Hospital in Tokyo, there were no gastric cancer–related deaths during a median follow-up period of 38 months (3–120 months). Although bleeding and perforation occurred in 5% of cases, there were no treatment-related deaths.[19] When perforation occurs, if immediately recognized, the problem can be fixed with intraluminal application of endoclips, and the risk of intraperitoneal seeding associated with such an event seems negligible.[31] For selected superficial T-1 cancers, EMR performed by experienced personnel can generate superb results and can be recommended, especially because any local recurrences can be addressed with salvage gastrectomy.

Laparoscopic resection with D1 lymphadenectomy and D1 pylorus-preserving gastrectomy represent valid options for T1 tumors not meeting EMR/ESR criteria.[24] However, for all T1 tumors meeting EMR/ESR criteria, this is probably the appropriate choice, because the risk of intra-abdominal seeding can be avoided and salvage for positive margin or for recurrence is feasible. The current Japanese treatment guidelines echo these views.[11]

EXTENT OF LYMPHADENECTOMY: D1 VERSUS D2

The Cape Town South Africa Trial (1982–1986)[32,33] of D1 versus D2 lymphadenectomy was conducted between 1/'82 and 11/'86, by Dent and colleagues[32] (this trial was termed Japanese R-1 vs Japanese R-2 at that time; the R term was subsequently replaced by the JGCA with D, to avoid confusion with the UICC R, a completeness-of-resection descriptor). Inclusion criteria included T1 to T3, N0 to N1 disease, no distant metastases, absence of significant comorbidity, and age less than 75 years. Patients from remote areas were excluded. For accurate staging, biopsies of celiac, common hepatic, and hepatic nodes and any abnormal nodes were taken for all patients. D2 (R-2 dissection in the nomenclature of the time) was performed according to the Japanese methods described by Kajitani[8]; specifically, removal of omentum, superior leaf of peritoneum on the transverse mesocolon, removal of the capsule of the pancreas (omentobursectomy, omental bursectomy, or bursectomy) and celiac-based lymph node dissection. For the gastric resection, gross proximal clearance of 5 cm was required in both arms, and reconstructive techniques were specified. During the period of study, 608 cases were reportedly evaluated, 403 were deemed surgical candidates, but only 43 (7% overall and 11% at laparotomy) were deemed to meet all eligibility criteria. Following treatment and discharge, patients were followed by examination at 3-month intervals. No attempt was made to screen for recurrence. No survival differences were noted. In-hospital mortality was zero for both groups. The trial did document increased operative time ($P<.005$), increased blood transfusions ($P<.005$) and longer hospital stay ($P<.05$) for the D2 group. This single-institution trial was halted when single-institution accrual was deemed insufficient to adequately power the study.[32,33]

The MRC Trial of Modified D1 versus Modified D2 Lymphadenectomy[34,35] was conducted from 1986 to 1995, by Cushieri and colleagues of the Surgical Cooperative Group. In this trial, a British D1 procedure was defined in a manner that was different from the definition used by the Japan Research Society for Gastric Cancer (JRSGC). For this trial, a D1 lymph node dissection was one in which only lymph nodes within 3 cm of the tumor were removed (consistent with older TNM definitions of N-1 nodes). The D2 procedure was defined as one in which TNM N-2 nodes (ie, celiac, hepatoduodenal, retroduodenal, splenic, and retropancreatic nodes, depending on the location of the tumor, as well as perigastric nodes >3 cm from the tumor) were removed and the omental bursa resected (omentobursectomy). Distal pancreaticosplenectomy was performed almost exclusively in the D2 group, and splenectomy in both groups, but more frequently in the D2 group. Eligibility was assessed at staging laparotomy. Prelaparotomy exclusions included age less than 20 years and those with serious comorbid disease. All patients were assessed at laparotomy for the presence of peritoneal implants, liver metastases, and extraregional/peri-aortic adenopathy, particularly in the area of the left renal vein. Patients with disease in these sites were excluded. Intraoperative peritoneal cytology was not used. Eligible cases were deemed to have TNM stage I to III disease with negative margins of resection and a proximal margin of at least 2.5 cm free of gross disease. Of 737 cases registered, 337 were deemed ineligible at staging laparotomy because of advanced disease, leaving 400 cases for intraoperative randomization. With median follow-up of 6.5 years, 5-year overall survival for the D1 group was 35% versus 33% for the D2 group (P = ns). Recurrence-free survival and disease-specific survival did not differ significantly. However, splenic resection, performed more frequently in the D2 group, and pancreatic resection, performed almost exclusively in the D2 group, seriously affected survival and proved to be independent predictors of poor survival. Complications and mortality were higher in the D2 group, and pancreaticosplenectomy was a powerful influence. The adverse impact of pancreaticosplenectomy, particularly pancreatectomy, confounded the lymphadenectomy question in this trial.[34,35]

The Dutch Trial of D1 versus D2 Lymphadenectomy[36–40] was conducted between August 1989 and July 1993 by surgeons participating in the Dutch Gastric Cancer Group. Eligibility criteria included age less than 85 years, adequate physical condition with no serious comorbid diseases, no previous cancer, no previous gastric surgery, and histologically confirmed gastric adenocarcinoma without evidence of distant metastases. Patients in both groups underwent distal or total gastrectomy according to the location of the tumor, with subtotal gastrectomy allowed if a proximal tumor-free margin of 5 cm could be achieved. At the onset of the trial, surgeons from 80 centers and 8 expert consulting surgeons were extensively instructed concerning Japanese-type surgical treatment according to JRSGC definitions and guidelines. Patients were randomized before surgery to arrange for the intraoperative presence of an expert consultant surgeon for all D2 cases. A Japanese expert surgeon attended every case during the first 4 months of the trial. The D1 procedure involved removal of all JRSGC-defined N1 nodes, generally the perigastric nodes at stations 1 to 6 along the greater and lesser curvatures of the stomach, along with removal of the lesser and greater omentum. The D2 procedure involved omentobursectomy (ie, removal of greater and lesser omentum, the superior leaf of the transverse mesocolon, and the capsule of the pancreas), frequent distal pancreatectomy and splenectomy (depending on tumor location), and removal of all JRSGC-defined N2 nodes at stations 7 to 12 (ie, left gastric, celiac, common hepatic, proper hepatic, and splenic artery, and splenic hilar nodes). Reconstruction following completion of the D2 node dissection was left to the local institutional surgeon, as was the postoperative care of the patient. Of the 1078 cases randomized before surgery, 82 (8%) were excluded for various reasons, most commonly unavailability of a consultant reference surgeon (35 cases), poor physical condition, or lack of histologic confirmation of the diagnosis. Of the remaining 996 patients randomized and entered into the study, 285 had evidence of incurable/extraregional disease at the time of surgery and were excluded. Seven-hundred and eleven deemed potentially curable underwent the randomly assigned treatment (ie, D1 or D2 resection) with curative intent. The 380 cases in the D1 group and the 331 cases in the D2 group were well balanced with respect to age, gender, tumor location, and tumor depth. Eighty-nine percent of the cases in each group were eventually shown to have undergone a pathologically confirmed, negative-margin, complete resection. A slightly higher proportion of cases in the D2 group underwent total gastrectomy (38% vs 30% in the D1 group). Among randomized cases, morbidity (25% vs 43%, P<.001) and in-hospital mortality (4% vs 10%, P = .004) were higher for the D2 group. With a median follow-up of 72 months,

5-year survival was 45% for the D1 group and 47% for the D2 group (P = ns).[37] Pancreatic and splenic resection, performed mostly in the D2 group (and mandated for particular tumor subsites) were associated with significantly higher morbidity and mortality in this study. Restricting the analysis to patients who did not undergo pancreatic or splenic resection (a post hoc, selected analysis), survival was higher for the D2 group (71% for the D2 group vs 59% for the D1 group, P = .02).[38] Overall, given the operations defined, those who had a negative-margin resection deemed potentially curative had a risk of relapse at 5 years of 43% for the D1 group compared with 37% for the D2 group (difference between relapse rates was not significant). An 11-year follow-on report for this trial indicated that, of the 89 cases in the trial with pathologic N2 disease, there were 9 survivors after 10 years, and that 8 of the 9 were in the D2 group (P = .01 for this post hoc analysis of the small N2 subgroup).[38] Overall survival at the 11-year mark is 31% versus 35% for D1 and D2 respectively (P = .53). A 2010 report with minimum 15-year follow-up on all patients clarifies that cumulative risk of death from gastric cancer is lower for the D2 group, but death from other causes is higher (**Fig. 2**). In the final analysis, there is no overall benefit to routine pre-1997 D2 lymphadenectomy when pancreas-spleen resection is a mandatory part of the operation for some tumors (**Fig. 3**).[40]

When the MRC trial and the Dutch trial were initiated, pancreaticosplenectomy was still deemed a standard part of a Japanese-type operation for cancers involving the cardia. By 1997, Japanese recommendations with respect to pancreaticosplenectomy had shifted,[41–43] but too late for these trials. Perhaps in response to MRC and Dutch trial findings, pancreas-preserving D2 operations are now considered standard, unless resection of these organs is required to achieve negative margins.[11,41–43]

Wu and colleagues[44] initiated a Taiwan trial of simple D1 lymphadenectomy versus enhanced celiac-based lymphadenectomy in 1993, before N-level definitions were changed in the 13th edition of the Japanese guidelines in 1997. What was previously defined by the Japanese as a D3 lymphadenectomy was redefined as a D2 lymphadenectomy in 1997. Although Wu and colleagues[44] state this fact in the introduction

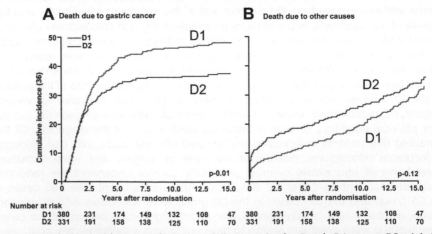

Fig. 2. Cumulative incidence, with 15-year follow-up, in the Dutch D1 versus D2 trial. (*A*) Death caused by gastric cancer; (*B*) death from other causes. N = 711. (*From* Songun I, Putter H, Kranenbarg EM, et al. Surgical treatment of gastric cancer: 15-year follow-up results of the randomised nationwide Dutch D1D2 trial. Lancet Oncol 2010;11(5):439–49; with permission.)

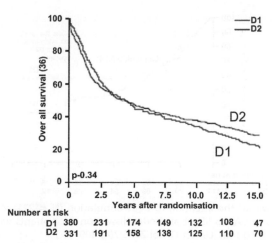

Fig. 3. Overall survival in the Dutch D1 versus D2 trial. (N = 711). (*From* Songun I, Putter H, Kranenbarg EM, et al. Surgical treatment of gastric cancer: 15-year follow-up results of the randomised nationwide Dutch D1D2 trial. Lancet Oncol 2010;11(5):439–49; with permission.)

to their article, their use of D3 in the title of the article has confused Western readers, who often overlook this study in their research into the D1 versus D2 question. To clarify terms, this article uses post-1997 definitions and identifies this as a D1 versus D2 trial. Conducted by 3 experienced expert surgeons at the Taipei Veterans General Hospital, who had each performed an audited series of 25 extended operations before any accrual was initiated, both follow-up (every 3 months with all follow-up conducted at the Taipei Veterans General Hospital) and quality control were meticulously monitored. Of 335 patients registered by August 1999, 221 patients (of median age 64.1 years) met prerandomization criteria and were randomized. The intraoperative randomization scheme used helped to minimize ineligible cases, but 64 cases were eventually found to not fit inclusion criteria, because of presence of T-1 (early) gastric cancer (54 patients), or microscopically positive margin of resection, positive peritoneal fluid cytology, or other reasons. There were 156 per protocol cases. The main analysis focused on the intent-to-treat population of 221 patients. Thirty-day surgical mortality was zero (0%) in both groups. As seen in **Fig. 4**, overall 5-year survival was 59.5% for the D3 group (D2 by current definitions) and 53.6% in the D1 group (log-rank $P = .041$). A Cox proportional hazards multivariate analysis, correcting for all prognostic variables, was also conducted and this also showed a lower hazard ratio for death in the more radically treated group (hazard ratio [HR] = 0.49, confidence interval [CI] 0.32–0.77, $P = .002$). Separate analysis of 156 per protocol cases (discussed earlier) revealed a 5-year survival of 51.3% for 76 D3 (currently defined as D2) cases and 45.0% for the 80 D1 cases (log-rank $P = .56$). A Cox proportional hazards multivariate analysis, correcting for all prognostic variables, was also conducted for this group, and this also showed lower HR for death in the more extensive lymphadenectomy group (HR = 0.42, $P = .0006$).[44,45]

Can a modern pancreas-preserving D2 operation be safely conducted in Western/European populations? To address this important question, Degiuli and colleagues[46,47] from 9 Italian institutions conducted a phase II trial from 1994 to 1996. Morbidity was 20.9% and in-hospital mortality was 3.1%, much lower than observed in the Dutch and MRC trials, in which a pancreas-preserving technique was not used. Five-year

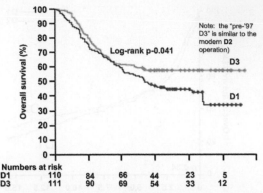

Fig. 4. Overall survival of the intention-to-treat population (N = 221) in the Taiwan trial. (*From* Wu CW, Hsiung CA, Lo SS, et al. Nodal dissection for patients with gastric cancer: a randomised controlled trial. Lancet Oncol 2006;7(4):309–15.)

survival in this study was 55%, comparable with the survival observed by Wu and colleagues.[46,47]

Summarizing these trial results (**Table 2**), for T2 to T4 gastric cancer, the modern, JGCA-defined, pancreas-preserving D2 operation is recommended, but only if it can be accomplished with minimal 30-day surgical mortality. Degiuli and colleagues[46,47] showed that this was possible in a European population, even in the mid-1990s. Throughout Asia today, 30-day surgical mortality for the D2 operation is generally less than 1%.[44,45,48,49] Today, throughout Asia, a pancreas-preserving D2 is considered the standard local-regional treatment of local-regional T2 to T4 gastric adenocarcinoma.[2,10,11]

For US and European populations (with more obesity as well as a greater burden of cardiovascular/cardiorespiratory comorbid disease), 30-day surgical mortality risk is generally higher. However, with reasonable patient selection Western experts can achieve Asian-like results with a pancreas-preserving D2 procedure.[46,47]

As discussed later, a customized pancreas-preserving Maruyama-guided lymphadenectomy can also generate superb results, and minimize potentially morbid overtreatment. Further, at least in the United States, in the event of surgical undertreatment (eg, a D0 or D1 lymphadenectomy, with higher risk of unresected regional disease), adjuvant postoperative chemoradiation is now routinely used. Particularly when the Maruyama Index of Unresected Disease" (MI) is high (ie, high risk of unresected nodal disease), most in the United States regard adjuvant chemoradiation as mandatory.[50,51] There is also some evidence that such adjuvant chemoradiation enhances survival after more adequate resection.[50,51]

MI AND PLANNING A LOW-MI OPERATION

In the late 1980s, Keiichi Maruyama and colleagues at the National Cancer Center Hospital in Tokyo created a useful computer program (known as the Maruyama Program), which searches a meticulously maintained 3843-patient database of gastric cancer cases treated by extensive lymphadenectomy (ie, D2 or more) for cases with characteristics similar to a given case. The program matches cases with similar characteristics, and reports observed nodal dissemination risk by individual lymph node station, as well as 5-year survival and other information. With 7 demographic and

Table 2
Purely surgical prospective randomized clinical trials: D1 versus D2 lymphadenectomy

Lymphadenectomy Trials	Inclusion Criteria	Mortality/Survival	Mortality/Survival	P Value (Survival)
		D1	D2	
Cape Town N = 43	T1-3; N0-1; M0 Age<75 y	0%/78% (3-y survival)	0%/76%	ns (3-y survival)
British MRC N = 400	Stage I–III Age>20 y	6%/35% (5-y survival)	13%/33%	ns (5-y survival)
Dutch N = 711	Stage I–II Age<85 y	4%/45% (5-y survival) 4%/21% (15 y survival)	10%/47% 10%/29%	ns(5-y survival) ns (15-y survival)
Taiwan N = 221 (intent to treat) N = 156 (per protocol)	No extraregional nodal disease No prior treatment Age≤75 y	0%/53.6% (5-y survival) 0%/45%	Pancreas-preserving D2 (ie, pre-1997 JGCA D3) 0%/59.5% 0%/51.3%	P = .041 (5-y survival) P = .056 (5-y survival)

Abbreviation: ns, not significant.

clinical inputs, all identifiable before or during surgery, the program predicts the statistical likelihood of nodal disease for each of the 16 main nodal stations around the stomach (ie, 12 main regional stations plus 4 main extraregional stations). Maruyama Program predictions have been assessed in Japanese, German, and Italian populations and found to be highly accurate.[52–54] The Maruyama Program is designed to be used by surgeons before or during surgery as a convenient means of rationally planning a data-driven lymphadenectomy for a given patient. Since the late 1980s, the program has been used in this way by many gastric cancer surgeons around the world. In an effort to expand the use of this computerized tool, a CD-ROM with expanded case volume was prepared in 2000.[55]

In a prospectively planned surgical analysis of a large adjuvant chemoradiation trial in the United States (the Macdonald Trail, SWOG 9008, Intergroup [INT] 0116), the extent of surgical treatment was specifically assessed and prospectively coded. The author designed a novel means of specifically quantifying the adequacy of lymphadenectomy relative to the likely extent of nodal disease for a given case, and termed this measure the MI. MI is defined as the sum of Maruyama Program predictions for Japanese-defined regional node stations (ie, stations 1–12) left in situ by the surgeon.[51] Based on the INT-0116 Macdonald trial's entry criteria, and the definition of MI, every case registered could have had an MI of zero. This variable was under the surgeon's control. As depicted in **Fig. 5**, median overall survival for the subgroup

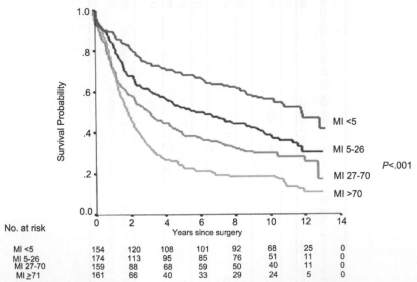

Fig. 5. Blinded reanalysis of the Dutch D1-D2 trial: overall survival and disease-free survival by MI quartiles. Survival by MI in the Dutch trial. Survival curves by MI quartiles reveal a strong dose-response effect. MI can be thought of as a quantitative yardstick for the adequacy of lymphadenectomy for a given case of gastric cancer. (*Data from* Peeters KC, Hundahl SA, Kranenbarg EK, et al. "Low-Maruyama-Index" surgery for gastric cancer - a blinded re-analysis of the Dutch D1-D2 trial. World J Surg 2005;29:1576–84; and Hundahl SA, Peeters KC, Kranenbarg EK, et al. Improved regional control and survival with "low Maruyama Index" surgery in gastric cancer: autopsy findings from the Dutch D1-D2 trial. Gastric Cancer 2007;10(2):84–6.)

with MI less than 5 (ie, those with a predicted risk of nodal disease left behind of less than 5%) was 91 months versus 27 months for others (P = .005). By multivariate analysis, adjusting for treatment, T-stage, and number of nodes positive, MI proved to be an independent predictor of both overall survival (P = .0049) and disease-free survival.[51,56] In addition, a dose-of-surgery effect, as measured by MI, was also evident: median survival was 20 months for the highest MI quartile and 46 months for the lowest MI quartile (treatment-adjusted P = .002).[51]

To further assess of the usefulness of MI as a prognostic tool, the Dutch D1 versus D2 trial was reanalyzed.[57] Blinded to survival, and eliminating cases with incomplete information, 648 of the 711 patients treated with curative intent had MI assigned. Median MI was 26 (ie, lower than the median MI of 70 in the Macdonald trial). Overall trial findings for D level were not affected by the absence of the 63 cases with incomplete data (ie, no overall survival difference between D1 and D2). In contrast with D level, and similar to findings as noted in the INT-0116 Macdonald chemoradiation trial, MI less than 5 proved a strong predictor of survival by both univariate and multivariate analysis (see **Fig. 5**). MI was an independent predictor of both overall survival (P = .016, HR = 1.45, 95% CI 1.07–1.95) and relapse risk (P = .010, HR = 1.72, 95% CI 1.14–2.60). Strong dose response with respect to MI and survival was also observed (see **Fig. 5**).[57] In addition, it has been shown by autopsy analysis of patients in the Dutch D1 to D2 trial that low-MI patients had less local and local-regional recurrence, but similar distant-disease recurrence.[58] The Dutch trial findings with respect to MI largely confirmed what was observed in the Macdonald trial.

The observed dose-response effect for MI suggests its use as a quantitative measure for the adequacy of lymphadenectomy in a given case of gastric cancer. As a quantitative measure, it can also identify patients at greater or lesser risk of local-regional recurrence. Whether or not to use this to influence decisions concerning postoperative adjuvant chemoradiotherapy remains controversial, because even low-MI cases may benefit. At a minimum, postresection MI data should be explicitly calculated and reported for every patient entered into a modern adjuvant trail.

Evidence in favor of the low-MI concept continues to emerge. For example, patients from a Dutch pre-CRITICS phase I/II chemoradiation trial have been matched with those in the Dutch D1 to D2 trial mentioned earlier. In this comparative analysis, low MI again proved to be a strong independent predictor of survival.[59]

EXTENDED PARA-AORTIC NODE DISSECTION (PRE-1997 D4 LYMPHADENECTOMY)

Several Japanese series document 5-year survival of 10% to 20% with successful resection of microscopic para-aortic lymph node metastases (M1 disease according to the UICC/AJCC TNM classification), particularly among patients with tumors in the proximal third of the stomach.[60–62] For patients with advanced gastric cancer at risk for such para-aortic disease, does routine resection of apparently uninvolved para-aortic nodes enhance survival?

From July, 1995 to April, 2001, the Japanese Clinical Oncology Group (JCOG) registered patients to JCOG9501, a prospective randomized trial of D2 plus extended para-aortic node dissection (the pre-1997 D4 operation). Investigators at participating institutions throughout Japan randomized 523 fit patients younger than 75 years of age with T2b-4 curable gastric cancer with no evidence of enlarged para-aortic nodes, negative peritoneal washing cytology, and no evidence of distant metastases to a modern D2 versus a pre-1997 D4 operation. To ensure fair balance, histologic assessment of para-aortic nodes during surgery was not allowed. In-hospital postoperative death was 0.8% in each group. Overall 5-year survival was 69.2% for the group assigned to D2 lymphadenectomy and 70.3% for the group assigned to D4 lympha-denectomy (log-rank P = .85). In a post hoc subgroup analysis, patients with histolog-ically node-negative disease had 5-year survival of 78.4% in the D2 group and 96.8% in the D4 group, a paradoxic result. Conversely, among node-positive patients, 5-year survival was 65.2% in the D2 group and 54.9% for patients in the D4 group, which is the opposite of the predicted result. Among the patients assigned to the para-aortic lymph node dissection group, HRs for death among the D4 para-aortic dissection group were 0.39 for the node-negative group and 1.39 for the node-positive group (P = .04). The investigators were unable to satisfactorily explain these paradoxic subgroup findings and have, in presentations, ruled out a data-coding error or detect-able occult disease in the negative nodes.[48,49]

A smaller, but otherwise identical, multicenter international trial was conducted from April 1995 to December 2002 by the East Asia Surgical Oncology Group. Centers in Japan, Korea, and Taiwan randomized 269 patients to D2 or D4 surgery. Eligibility criteria were similar to those of the JCOG trial described earlier. In this trial, 5-year survival was 52.6% for the group assigned to D2 lymphadenectomy and 55.0% among the group assigned to D4 lymphadenectomy (P = .801).[63]

Based on these trial findings (**Table 3**), routine para-aortic lymphadenectomy is not recommended.

FUTURE TRIALS

Presently (2011) throughout the world, adjuvant or neoadjuvant systemic chemo-therapy, and/or chemoradiotherapy, have become commonplace for advanced (ie, T2–T4) gastric cancer.[11,64–67] Although surgical questions will continue to be built into adjuvant and neoadjuvant trials for advanced gastric cancer, the trials dis-cussed earlier probably represent the final answer with respect to purely surgical trials concerning the regional lymphadenectomy question and the extent-of-resection question. However, some forthcoming trials of other surgical questions deserve mention.

Omental bursectomy (aka omentobursectomy) involves en-bloc resection of both the anterior capsule of the pancreas and the (continuous) superior leaf of

Table 3					
Prospective randomized clinical trials: extended para-aortic node dissection (pre-1997 JGCA D4)					
Total vs Subtotal Trials		Inclusion Criteria	Mortality/ Survival	Mortality/ Survival	P Value (Survival)
			D2	D4	
Sasako et al[22,48,49,65]	N = 523	T2b–T4 tumor Age<75 y No adjuvant therapy No gross para-aortic disease	0.8%/69.2% vs	8%/70.3%	0.85 (ns)
			D2	D4	
Yonemura et al[63]	N = 293	T2–T4 tumor Age<75 y No adjuvant therapy No gross para-aortic disease	0.74%/52.6% vs	3.7%/55.0%	0.80 (ns)

Abbreviation: ns, not significant.

peritoneum on the transverse mesocolon. In this way, the floor of the omental bursa is removed with the surgical specimen. Surgeons often include this as part of a Japanese-style gastrectomy for cancer and this maneuver greatly facilitates complete removal of the (very high-risk) station 6 subpyloric lymph nodes. For sub-serosal or serosal tumors on the posterior wall of the stomach, local peritoneal implants neighboring the tumor can be entirely resected by this maneuver. Hydro-dissection, with saline injection beneath the peritoneal layer, can greatly facilitate this maneuver, particularly during initial attempts. Does this have oncologic value or can this surgical maneuver be eliminated? A pilot study in Japan, designed to show that elimination of omental bursectomy was acceptable in terms of survival, documented the opposite. Between July 2002 and January 2007, a total of 210 patients at Osaka hospitals were randomized to either the bursectomy group or to the nonbursectomy group. Background characteristics, blood loss, and so forth were well balanced. Overall morbidity was equal in both groups (14%), and the in-hospital mortality was equal (0.95%) in both groups. In the first interim analysis, the 3-year overall survival was 86% in the bursectomy group and 79% in the nonbur-sectomy group, with an HR of 1.55 (95% CI 0.84–2.84). The nonbursectomy group had more patients with peritoneal recurrences than the bursectomy group (14% vs 8%). Among the 48 cases with pT3 or T4 disease, 3 year overall survival was 69.8% for the bursectomy group and 50.2% for the non-bursectomy group (HR for death 2.16 for the non-bursectomy group; p value = ns).[68] From early results of this non-inferiority study, a larger, better-powered JCOG trial (JCOG1001), examining the potential value of omental bursectomy during D2 resection of subserosal and trans-serosal posterior gastric tumors, is being initiated.[11]

For patients with advanced proximal third tumors along the greater curvature of the stomach, routine splenectomy for clearance of lymph node station 10 nodes (at the splenic hilum) is being investigated in JCOG0110.[11,69]

Among patients with unresectable metastatic disease, the potential survival and palliative value of surgical debulking is being explored. The so-called REGATTA Trial (JCOG0705 and KGCA-01) has been initiated to explore this issue.[11,70]

SUMMARY

For selected T1 cancers unlikely to be associated with nodal disease, ESR offers excellent results without the morbidity and risk of major surgery. For recurrences after EMR or ESR, salvage treatment with completion gastrectomy is possible.

For T2 to T4 cancers, negative-margin (R-0) resection is to be achieved by distal subtotal gastrectomy whenever feasible. The pancreas and spleen should be preserved unless invaded. Lymphadenectomy can be customized by preoperative or intraoperative use of the Maruyama Program to generate a low-MI operation. This potentially minimizes perioperative morbidity and mortality by restricting nodal dissection to at-risk node stations likely to harbor disease. After surgery, the compel-ling dose-response effect for MI suggests its use as a quantitative measure for the adequacy of lymphadenectomy. Using this measure to select patients for adjuvant chemoradiation may have merit, but this question has not been specifically answered.

For local-regional T2 to T4 disease resectable to negative margins, a JGCA-defined pancreas-preserving D2 operation is also appropriate, provided this can be accom-plished with low 30-day mortality risk. As noted, most Asian centers are now reporting risk of 1% or less.

Although surgical resection of microscopic disease in para-aortic nodes can be associated with prolonged disease-free survival in up to 10% to 20% of cases, prospective randomized trials have shown no advantage to routine para-aortic node dissection, and this cannot be recommended.

With regard to future and pending trials, the value of omental bursectomy, of splenectomy for selected tumors, and of (reduction surgery by) debulking are all being investigated.

REFERENCES

1. Schlemper RJ, Riddell RH, Kato Y, et al. The Vienna classification of gastrointestinal epithelial neoplasia. Gut 2000;47(2):251–5.
2. Japanese Gastric Cancer Association. Japanese classification of gastric carcinoma: 3rd English edition. Gastric Cancer 2011;14(2):101–12.
3. Ho CL. Clinical PET imaging–an Asian perspective. Ann Acad Med Singapore 2004;33(2):155–65.
4. Mochiki E, Kuwano H, Katoh H, et al. Evaluation of 18F-2-deoxy-2-fluoro-D-glucose positron emission tomography for gastric cancer. World J Surg 2004; 28(3):247–53.
5. Stahl A, Ott K, Weber WA, et al. FDG PET imaging of locally advanced gastric carcinomas: correlation with endoscopic and histopathological findings. Eur J Nucl Med Mol Imaging 2003;30(2):288–95.
6. Edge SB, Compton CC, Fritz AG, et al. AJCC cancer staging manual. 7th edition. New York: Springer; 2009.
7. Sobin L, Gospodarowicz M, Wittekind. TNM Classification of Malignant Tumors. Seventh Edition. Indianapolis: Wiley-Blackwell; 2009.
8. Kajitani T. The general rules for the gastric cancer study in surgery and pathology. Part I. Clinical classification. Jpn J Surg 1981;11(2):127–39.
9. Sayegh ME, Sano T, Dexter S, et al. TNM and Japanese staging systems for gastric cancer: how do they coexist? Gastric Cancer 2004;7(3):140–8.
10. Sano T, Aiko T. New Japanese classifications and treatment guidelines for gastric cancer: revision concepts and major revised points. Gastric Cancer 2011;14(2): 97–100.
11. Japanese Gastric Cancer Association. Japanese gastric cancer treatment guidelines 2010 (ver. 3). Gastric Cancer 2011;14(2):113–23.
12. Gouzi JL, Huguier M, Fagniez PL, et al. Total versus subtotal gastrectomy for adenocarcinoma of the gastric antrum. A French prospective controlled study. Ann Surg 1989;209(2):162–6.
13. McNeer G, Pack G. Neoplasms of the Stomach. Philadelphia: Lippincott; 1967.
14. McNeer G, Bowden L, Booner RJ, et al. Elective total gastrectomy for cancer of the stomach: end results. Ann Surg 1974;180(2):252–6.
15. Bozzetti F. Surgical treatment of Borrmann type IV gastric carcinoma. J Am Coll Surg 1997;185(2):200–1.
16. Bozzetti F, Marubini E, Bonfanti G, et al. Subtotal versus total gastrectomy for gastric cancer: five-year survival rates in a multicenter randomized Italian trial. Italian Gastrointestinal Tumor Study Group. Ann Surg 1999;230(2):170–8.
17. Bozzetti F, Marubini E, Bonfanti G, et al. Total versus subtotal gastrectomy: surgical morbidity and mortality rates in a multicenter Italian randomized trial. The Italian Gastrointestinal Tumor Study Group. Ann Surg 1997;226(5): 613–20.
18. Robertson CS, Chung SC, Woods SD, et al. A prospective randomized trial comparing R1 subtotal gastrectomy with R3 total gastrectomy for antral cancer. Ann Surg 1994;220(2):176–82.

19. Ono H, Kondo H, Gotoda T, et al. Endoscopic mucosal resection for treatment of early gastric cancer. Gut 2001;48(2):225–9.
20. Pathirana A, Poston GJ. Lessons from Japan–endoscopic management of early gastric and oesophageal cancer. Eur J Surg Oncol 2001;27(1):9–16.
21. Sano T, Katai H, Sasako M, et al. The management of early gastric cancer. Surg Oncol 2000;9(1):17–22.
22. Sasako M. Treatment of early gastric cancer. Chir Ital 1997;49(3):9–13.
23. Hiki Y. [Endoscopic mucosal resection (EMR) for early gastric cancer.] Nippon Geka Gakkai Zasshi 1996;97(4):273–8 [in Japanese].
24. Kobayashi T, Kazui T, Kimura T. Surgical local resection for early gastric cancer. Surg Laparosc Endosc Percutan Tech 2003;13(5):299–303.
25. Yamamoto H, Sekine Y, Higashizawa T, et al. Successful en bloc resection of a large superficial gastric cancer by using sodium hyaluronate and electrocautery incision forceps. Gastrointest Endosc 2001;54(5):629–32.
26. Yoshikane H, Sakakibara A, Hidano H, et al. Piecemeal endoscopic aspiration mucosectomy for large superficial intramucosal tumors of the stomach. Endoscopy 2001;33(9):795–9.
27. Kobayashi T, Gotohda T, Tamakawa K, et al. Magnetic anchor for more effective endoscopic mucosal resection. Jpn J Clin Oncol 2004;34(3):118–23.
28. Gotoda T, Oda I, Tamakawa K, et al. Prospective clinical trial of magnetic-anchor-guided endoscopic submucosal dissection for large early gastric cancer (with videos). Gastrointest Endosc 2009;69(1):10–5.
29. Kuwano H, Mochiki E, Asao T, et al. Double endoscopic intraluminal operation for upper digestive tract diseases: proposal of a novel procedure. Ann Surg 2004; 239(1):22–7.
30. Gotoda T, Yanagisawa A, Sasako M, et al. Incidence of lymph node metastasis from early gastric cancer: estimation with a large number of cases at two large centers. Gastric Cancer 2000;3(4):219–25.
31. Ikehara H, Gotoda T, Ono H, et al. Gastric perforation during endoscopic resection for gastric carcinoma and the risk of peritoneal dissemination. Br J Surg 2007;94(8):992–5.
32. Dent DM, Madden MV, Price SK. Randomized comparison of R1 and R2 gastrectomy for gastric carcinoma. Br J Surg 1988;75(2):110–2.
33. Dent DM. Radical surgery for curable gastric carcinoma. S Afr Med J 1994;84(2): 56–7.
34. Cuschieri A, Fayers P, Fielding J, et al. Postoperative morbidity and mortality after D1 and D2 resections for gastric cancer: preliminary results of the MRC randomised controlled surgical trial. The Surgical Cooperative Group. Lancet 1996; 347(9007):995–9.
35. Cuschieri A, Weeden S, Fielding J, et al. Patient survival after D1 and D2 resections for gastric cancer: long- term results of the MRC randomized surgical trial. Surgical Co-operative Group. Br J Cancer 1999;79(9–10):1522–30.
36. Bonenkamp JJ, Songun I, Hermans J, et al. Randomised comparison of morbidity after D1 and D2 dissection for gastric cancer in 996 Dutch patients. Lancet 1995; 345(8952):745–8.
37. Bonenkamp JJ, Hermans J, Sasako M, et al. Extended lymph-node dissection for gastric cancer. Dutch Gastric Cancer Group. N Engl J Med 1999;340(12): 908–14.
38. Hartgrink HH, Van De Velde CJ, Putter H, et al. Extended Lymph node dissection for gastric cancer: who may benefit? Final results of the Randomized Dutch Gastric Cancer Group Trial. J Clin Oncol 2004;22:2069–77.

39. Hartgrink HH, van de Velde CJ. Status of extended lymph node dissection: locoregional control is the only way to survive gastric cancer. J Surg Oncol 2005;90(3):153–65.
40. Songun I, Putter H, Kranenbarg EM, et al. Surgical treatment of gastric cancer: 15-year follow-up results of the randomised nationwide Dutch D1D2 trial. Lancet Oncol 2010;11(5):439–49.
41. Maruyama K, Sasako M, Kinoshita T, et al. Pancreas-preserving total gastrectomy for proximal gastric cancer. World J Surg 1995;19(4):532–6.
42. Uyama I, Ogiwara H, Takahara T, et al. Spleen- and pancreas-preserving total gastrectomy with superextended lymphadenectomy including dissection of the para-aortic lymph nodes for gastric cancer. J Surg Oncol 1996;63(4):268–70.
43. Kaminishi M, Shimoyama S, Yamaguchi H, et al. Results of subtotal gastrectomy with complete dissection of the N2 lymph nodes preserving the spleen and pancreas in surgery for gastric cancer. Hepatogastroenterology 1994;41(4):384–7.
44. Wu CW, Hsiung CA, Lo SS, et al. Nodal dissection for patients with gastric cancer: a randomised controlled trial. Lancet Oncol 2006;7(4):309–15.
45. Wu CW, Chang IS, Lo SS, et al. Complications following D3 gastrectomy: post hoc analysis of a randomized trial. World J Surg 2006;30(1):12–6.
46. Degiuli M, Sasako M, Ponti A, et al. Survival results of a multicentre phase II study to evaluate D2 gastrectomy for gastric cancer. Br J Cancer 2004;90(9):1727–32.
47. Degiuli M, Sasako M, Ponti A, et al. Morbidity and mortality after D2 gastrectomy for gastric cancer: results of the Italian Gastric Cancer Study Group prospective multicenter surgical study. J Clin Oncol 1998;16(4):1490–3.
48. Sasako M, Sano S, Yamamoto A, et al. Randomized phase III trial of standard D2 versus D2 + para-aortic lymph node (PAN) dissection (D) for clinically M0 advanced gastric cancer: JCOG9501. J Clin Oncol 2006;24(18-s, part II):934-s.
49. Sasako M, Sano T, Yamamoto S, et al. D2 lymphadenectomy alone or with para-aortic nodal dissection for gastric cancer. N Engl J Med 2008;359(5):453–62.
50. Macdonald JS, Smalley SR, Benedetti J, et al. Chemoradiotherapy after surgery compared with surgery alone for adenocarcinoma of the stomach or gastro-esophageal junction. N Engl J Med 2001;345(10):725–30.
51. Hundahl SA, Macdonald JS, Benedetti J, et al. Surgical treatment variation in a prospective, randomized trial of chemoradiotherapy in gastric cancer: the effect of undertreatment. Ann Surg Oncol 2002;9(3):278–86.
52. Kampschoer GH, Maruyama K, van de Velde CJ, et al. Computer analysis in making preoperative decisions: a rational approach to lymph node dissection in gastric cancer patients. Br J Surg 1989;76(9):905–8.
53. Bollschweiler E, Boettcher K, Hoelscher AH, et al. Preoperative assessment of lymph node metastases in patients with gastric cancer: evaluation of the Maruyama computer program. Br J Surg 1992;79(2):156–60.
54. Guadagni S, de Manzoni G, Catarci M, et al. Evaluation of the Maruyama computer program accuracy for preoperative estimation of lymph node metastases from gastric cancer. World J Surg 2000;24(12):1550–8.
55. Siewert JR, Kelsen D, Maruyama K, et al. Gastric cancer diagnosis and treatment - an interactive training program, vol. 2000. Heidelberg (for Germans) and New York: Springer Electronic Media; 2000.
56. Hundahl SA, Macdonald JS, Benedetti J. Durable survival impact of "Low Maruyama Index Surgery" in a trial of adjuvant chemoradiation for gastric

cancer. Alexandria (VA): American Society of Clinical Oncology, 2004 ASCO GI Symposium; 2004.

57. Peeters KC, Hundahl SA, Kranenbarg EK, et al. "Low-Maruyama-Index" surgery for gastric cancer - a blinded re-analysis of the Dutch D1-D2 trial. World J Surg 2005;29:1576-84.

58. Hundahl SA, Peeters KC, Kranenbarg EK, et al. Improved regional control and survival with "low Maruyama Index" surgery in gastric cancer: autopsy findings from the Dutch D1-D2 trial. Gastric Cancer 2007;10(2):84-6.

59. Dikken JL, Jansen EP, Cats A, et al. Impact of the extent of surgery and postoperative chemoradiotherapy on recurrence patterns in gastric cancer. J Clin Oncol 2010;28(14):2430-6.

60. Baba M, Hokita S, Natsugoe S, et al. Paraaortic lymphadenectomy in patients with advanced carcinoma of the upper-third of the stomach. Hepatogastroenterology 2000;47(33):893-6.

61. Isozaki H, Okajima K, Fujii K, et al. Effectiveness of paraaortic lymph node dissection for advanced gastric cancer. Hepatogastroenterology 1999;46(25):549-54.

62. Maeta M, Saito H, Cai J, et al. Immunohistochemical detection of occult metastases in paraaortic lymph nodes in advanced gastric cancer. Oncol Rep 1999;6(6):1233-6.

63. Yonemura Y, Wu CC, Fukushima N, et al. Randomized clinical trial of D2 and extended paraaortic lymphadenectomy in patients with gastric cancer. Int J Clin Oncol 2008;13(2):132-7.

64. Cunningham D, Allum WH, Stenning SP, et al. Perioperative chemotherapy versus surgery alone for resectable gastroesophageal cancer. N Engl J Med 2006;355(1):11-20.

65. Sasako M, Saka M, Fukagawa T, et al. [Adjuvant chemotherapy using S-1 for curatively resected gastric cancer-the nationwide clinical trial.] Gan To Kagaku Ryoho 2006;33(Suppl 1):110-6 [in Japanese].

66. Sakuramoto S, Sasako M, Yamaguchi T, et al. Adjuvant chemotherapy for gastric cancer with S-1, an oral fluoropyrimidine. N Engl J Med 2007;357(18):1810-20.

67. Jansen EP, Boot H, Dubbelman R, et al. Postoperative chemoradiotherapy in gastric cancer-a phase I-II study of radiotherapy with dose escalation of weekly cisplatin and daily capecitabine chemotherapy. Ann Oncol 2010;21(3):530-4.

68. Fujita J, Kurokawa Y, Sugimoto T, et al. Survival benefit of bursectomy in patients with resectable gastric cancer: interim analysis results of a randomized controlled trial. Gastric Cancer 2011 May 15. [Epub ahead of print].

69. Sano T, Yamamoto S, Sasako M. Randomized controlled trial to evaluate splenectomy in total gastrectomy for proximal gastric carcinoma: Japan Clinical Oncology Group Study JCOG 0110-MF. Jpn J Clin Oncol 2002;32(9):363-4.

70. Fujitani K, Yang HK, Kurokawa Y, et al. Randomized controlled trial comparing gastrectomy plus chemotherapy with chemotherapy alone in advanced gastric cancer with a single non-curable factor: Japan Clinical Oncology Group Study JCOG 0705 and Korea Gastric Cancer Association Study KGCA01. Jpn J Clin Oncol 2008;38(7):504-6.

Preoperative and Postoperative Chemotherapy for Gastric Cancer

Vikram K. Jain, FRACP, David Cunningham, MD, Ian Chau, MD*

KEYWORDS

• Gastric cancer • Chemotherapy • Operable

Gastric cancer is the second leading cause of death from malignancy,[1] with approximately 989,600 new cases and more than 738,000 deaths occurring every year worldwide.[2] A significant geographic variation exists, with the highest rates reported in East Asia, South America, and Eastern Europe. In the Western world, gastric cancer is often diagnosed at an advanced stage in the majority of the patients, in contrast to Japan where the use of screening enables detection of early disease. Although the overall incidence of gastric cancer is decreasing,[3] there has been a relative increase in the incidence of tumors of the gastroesophageal junction (GOJ) and the gastric cardia,[4] thought to be a consequence of rising levels of obesity and gastroesophageal reflux disease.[5] Multimodality therapy using chemotherapy, radiation, or a combination of both has demonstrated improved outcomes in comparison with surgery alone; however, a marked variation is seen in different parts of the world with regard to timing, sequence, and treatment modality used. In East Asia, D2 surgical dissection is followed by adjuvant oral fluoropyrimidine-based therapy, whereas a perioperative approach with chemotherapy given before and after surgery is followed in Europe. By contrast, in the United States adjuvant chemoradiation is commonly used following curative surgery in patients with gastric cancer. In this review the authors discuss the role of chemotherapy in the preoperative and postoperative management of gastric cancer, and suggest various approaches for the integration of systemic chemotherapy into the treatment paradigm.

Conflicts of interest: Dr Vikram K. Jain has no conflicts of interest: Dr Ian Chau has received research funding from Roche, Novartis, and Merck Serono, and has a consultant/advisory role for Roche, Novartis, Merck Sereno, and Imclone. Prof Cunningham has received research funding from Amgen, Roche, Merck Sharpe and Dohme, Sanofi-Aventis, and Merck Serono, and has participated in uncompensated advisory boards for Roche and Amgen.
Department of Medicine, Royal Marsden Hospital, Down's Road, Sutton, Surrey SM2 5PT, UK
* Corresponding author.
E-mail address: Ian.Chau@rmh.nhs.uk

RATIONALE FOR CHEMOTHERAPEUTIC STRATEGIES IN GASTRIC CANCER

Despite radical surgery, most patients undergoing curative resection relapse with local and systemic recurrence, leading to poor overall survival. This recurrence is most likely due to occult metastatic disease in the tumor bed and distant sites, hence multimodality approaches using chemotherapy, radiation, or a combination of both have been evaluated in last few decades in an attempt to improve outcomes following surgery. Regardless of the differences that exist amongst these approaches, a benefit is usually seen from adding systemic chemotherapy, thereby reinforcing the concept that operable gastric cancer is in fact a local presentation of a systemic disease that has occult micrometastatic disease at the time of diagnosis, leading to relapse and poor survival after radical surgery.

TREATMENT PLANNING AND SURGERY

A multidisciplinary team approach, comprising surgeons, medical and radiation oncologists, gastroenterologists, radiologists, and pathologists is required for the optimal management of patients with gastric cancer. Size and location of the tumor influence the choice of treatment. Surgical resection of the primary tumor and regional lymph nodes is a key step in the curative treatment of gastric cancer. The extent of resection is determined by the preoperative stage. Endoscopic mucosal resection (EMR) is being increasingly offered to patients with cancer limited to mucosa, which is 2 cm or smaller and histologically well differentiated with no evidence of ulceration.[6] Annual endoscopic surveillance is necessary after EMR to exclude local recurrence and metachronous gastric cancer. The incidence of lymph node involvement increases up to 20% in the tumors involving submucosa, and these patients require gastrectomy with lymph node dissection. Radical gastrectomy is indicated for patients with disease of stage 1b to III. Whereas a total gastrectomy is done for proximal tumors, a subtotal gastrectomy can be performed for distal tumors, providing a macroscopic proximal margin of 5 cm can be achieved between the tumor and the GOJ. The extent of lymphadenectomy D1 (removal of perigastric lymph nodes) versus D2 (removal of perigastric lymph nodes plus those along the celiac axis and left gastric, common hepatic, and splenic arteries) dissection during gastrectomy for gastric cancer has been a matter of great controversy. Although D2 lymphadenectomy is frequently practiced in Japan and East Asia; data from two large randomized trials conducted in the West have so far failed to demonstrate superiority of D2 dissection over D1.[7,8] Long-term follow-up results from the Dutch trial[9] demonstrated a significantly lower locoregional recurrence and gastric cancer–related death (15-year gastric cancer-specific survival 48% vs 37%, $P = .01$) with D2 resection; however, similar to previous data, no significant improvement in overall survival (28% vs 22%, $P = .34$) was demonstrated. Extended lymphadenectomy with pancreas and spleen preservation (known as "over D1") is often practiced in Western countries, as it allows more precise tumor staging and postoperative treatment planning.

ADJUVANT STRATEGIES

Due to high rates of local and systemic recurrence after curative surgical resection and subsequent poor survival, multiple studies have evaluated strategies using chemotherapy, radiotherapy, or a combination of both in the adjuvant setting to improve patient outcomes. Adjuvant radiotherapy alone has failed to achieve a survival benefit for patients with gastric cancer[10]; however, a survival benefit has been demonstrated from the addition of chemoradiation or chemotherapy in the adjuvant setting.

Adjuvant Chemoradiation

Encouraging effects on local control and survival were demonstrated in early-phase studies that evaluated chemoradiation in patients with localized gastric cancer **Table 1**.[11,12] Based on this, the larger phase 3 US Intergroup 0116 Study[13] randomly assigned 556 patients following curative resection of gastric cancer (stage 1b–IV) to observation alone or adjuvant chemoradiotherapy. Adjuvant treatment consisted of 5 monthly cycles of bolus chemotherapy with 5-fluorouracil (5-FU) and leucovorin daily for 5 days with radiotherapy given concurrently with cycles 2 and 3 (**Table 1**).

After 5 years of follow-up, the median overall survival was significantly longer after chemoradiation than after surgery alone (36 months vs 27 months; P = .005), and a marked benefit was also seen in progression-free survival (hazard ratio [HR] 1.52; 95% confidence interval [CI] 1.23–1.86; P<.001). Updated results with more than 10-year median follow-up also demonstrated continued benefit from the chemoradiation with overall survival (HR = 1.32; P = .004) and disease-free survival (HR 1.51; P<.001) favoring chemoradiation.[14] Although this trial led to adjuvant chemoradiation being adopted as a standard therapy for patients with curatively resected gastric cancer in the United States, it has not gained worldwide acceptance because of concerns about the quality of surgery used and the toxicity of abdominal chemoradiation. In both arms the patients had high risk of relapse following surgery (more than two-thirds of patients had T3 or T4 tumors and 85% had positive lymph nodes), but most patients had what is considered a suboptimal surgery (54% had only D0 resection). The effects of the inadequate surgery were probably counterbalanced by adjuvant treatment in the chemoradiation arm,[15] although in an update in 2004 no difference in treatment effect by the level of surgery performed was reported.[16]

The recently presented CALGB 80101[17] trial assessed the benefit of using combination chemotherapy with epirubicin, cisplatin, and 5-FU (ECF) with postoperative chemoradiation in patients with resected adenocarcinoma of the stomach or GOJ. No benefit was demonstrated with the use of ECF chemotherapy before and after 5-FU chemoradiation in comparison with bolus 5-FU/leucovorin given before and after 5-FU/radiotherapy. However, this trial used only one cycle of full-dose ECF regimen

Table 1
Major practice-changing phase 3 trials in operable gastric cancer

Trial Name	Intervention	No. of Patients	5-Year Overall Survival	Hazard Ratio (95% Confidence Intervals), P Value
Intergroup 0116[14]	Surgery	277	41%	1.31 (1.09–1.59)
	Surgery + adjuvant 5-FU/LV chemoradiation	282	50%	P = .005
MAGIC[36]	Surgery	250	23.0%	0.75 (0.60–0.93)
	Perioperative chemotherapy + surgery	253	36.3%	P = .009
FFCD[37]	Surgery	111	24%	0.69 (0.50–0.95)
	Perioperative chemotherapy + surgery	113	38%	P = .003
ACTS-GC[32]	Observation	530	61.4%	0.65 (0.53–0.81)
	Adjuvant S-1	529	72.6%	

Abbreviations: 5-FU, 5-fluorouracil; LV, leucovorin.

before chemoradiation and 2 cycles of dose-attenuated ECF were given post chemo-radiation, thereby making it difficult to draw any conclusions regarding the benefit or lack of benefit from the addition of triplet chemotherapy. Of interest, the median 3-year survival in the CALGB study[17] was almost identical to that of the Intergroup 0116[13] trial, which was conducted more than 10 years ago. At present, quality control data for surgery are not available to assess the quality of surgery, which was the subject of much criticism of the Intergroup 0116[13] trial.

Whether adjuvant radiation is beneficial after optimal gastric surgery (D2 resection or higher) has been a matter of great controversy. In retrospective analyses, a benefit from adjuvant chemoradiation after surgery, and even after D2 resection, has been suggested.[18,19] The role of adjuvant radiation after D2 resection will be evaluated prospectively by the randomized phase 3 Korean ARTIST[20] study, which recently completed accrual of 458 patients after surgery to adjuvant cisplatin and capecitabine or cisplatin/capecitabine chemoradiation (see **Table 2**). Also, the ongoing phase 3 CRITICS trial will evaluate the benefits of adding postoperative chemoradiation to perioperative ECX (epirubicin, cisplatin, capecitabine) combination chemotherapy. Nevertheless, at present postoperative chemoradiation remains one of the standard options for treatment of patients with curatively resected gastric cancer, and is widely used in the United States.

Adjuvant Chemotherapy

Over the last 30 years, multiple randomized studies have evaluated the role of adjuvant chemotherapy in gastric cancer. Unfortunately, many of these were underpowered for survival and often used "suboptimal" regimens, with consequent variable results. The

Table 2
Selected ongoing trials in gastric cancer

Trial Name	Eligible Population	Planned Recruitment	Treatment Arms
ARTIST	Resected stage Ib–IV gastric cancer (D2 or higher resection)	458 (completed recruitment)	Adjuvant ECF chemoradiation Adjuvant CX Adjuvant CX chemoradiation
CRITICS	Stage Ib–IV gastric cancer	788	Perioperative ECX chemotherapy before and after surgery Preoperative ECX chemotherapy then adjuvant CX chemoradiation
SAMIT	T3/T4 gastric carcinoma	1495 (completed recruitment)	Adjuvant UFT for 11 months Adjuvant S-1 for 11 months Adjuvant paclitaxel for 3 months, then adjuvant UFT for 8 months Adjuvant paclitaxel for 3 months, then UFT for 8 months
ST03	Stage Ib–IV resectable adenocarcinoma of the stomach or GOJ	950	Perioperative ECX 3 cycles before and 3 after surgery Perioperative ECX + bevacizumab 3 cycles before and after surgery, then maintenance bevacizumab for 6 cycles

Abbreviations: CX, cisplatin, capecitabine; ECF, epirubicin, cisplatin, continuous-infusion 5-fluoro-uracil; ECX, epirubicin, cisplatin, capecitabine; GOJ, gastroesophageal junction; UFT, uracil/tegafur.

majority of these trials were conducted in East Asia, with only two small randomized trials conducted in the West demonstrating a survival benefit from adjuvant chemo-therapy.[21,22] Although until the late 1990s adjuvant chemotherapy was generally not considered to be of benefit in operable gastric cancer,[23] a survival benefit, albeit small, was demonstrated on subsequent meta-analyses that were conducted to evaluate to role of adjuvant chemotherapy in gastric cancer.[24–28] Recently, a large individual patient-level meta-analysis containing data from 17 randomized controlled trials (n = 3838) demonstrated significantly improved overall survival from postoperative adjuvant 5-FU–based chemotherapy when compared with surgery alone (55.3% vs 49.6%; HR 0.82; 95% CI 0.76–0.90; $P<.001$). No significant heterogeneity across randomized studies or for the choice of chemotherapy regimen used was reported in this meta-analysis.[29]

Among randomized studies of adjuvant chemotherapy in gastric cancer, perhaps most intriguing are results of the two recent trials conducted in East Asia, the ACTS-GC[30] and the CLASSIC[31] study, which evaluated the role of chemotherapy after D2 resection surgery. The ACTS-GC[30] study, a Japanese adjuvant trial, randomized 1059 patients with stage II or III D2 resected gastric cancer to observation, or 1 year's treatment with adjuvant S-1 chemotherapy. S-1 is an orally active combination of tegafur (5-fluorouracil prodrug), gimeracil (an inhibitor of dihydropyrimidine dehydro-genase, which degrades fluorouracil), and oteracil (inhibits phosphorylation of fluoro-uracil in the gastrointestinal tract) in a molar ratio of 1:0.4:1. The trial, which was stopped early because of positive efficacy results at interim analysis, demonstrated a significant 10% improvement in 3-year overall survival from adjuvant S-1 chemotherapy after surgery (80.1% vs 70.1%; $P = .002$). Updated results with longer follow-up have also confirmed the benefit of adjuvant S-1, with nearly 11% improve-ment in 5-year overall survival compared with surgery alone (72.6% vs 61.4%; HR 0.65; 95% CI 0.53–0.81).[32] Most recently, a Korean study, the phase 3 CLASSIC[31] study (n = 1035), reported a significant benefit in disease-free survival (DFS) from adjuvant combination chemotherapy. Following D2 resection, patients with stage II, IIIa, and IIIb gastric cancer were randomized to adjuvant CAPOX (capecitabine 1000 mg/m^2 twice a day days 1–14 every 3 weeks, and oxaliplatin 130 mg/m^2 day 1, every 3 weeks × 8 cycles) or observation alone. Although the data analysis was planned after 385 DFS events had occurred, the independent data-monitoring committee recommended a full evaluation and reporting of results following a signifi-cant preplanned interim analysis at 266 events. Patients treated with adjuvant XELOX had significantly improved 3-year DFS compared with the surgery-alone arm (74% vs 60%; HR 0.56; 95% CI 0.44–0.72; $P<.0001$) with a trend toward improved overall survival (HR 0.74; 95% CI 0.53–1.03; $P = .0775$), although the data were still immature for analysis of overall survival at this point. Data from both the ACTS-GC and CLASSIC study confirm that even after "optimal" (D-2) gastric resection surgery, there is a benefit to be gained from the use of adjuvant chemotherapy. Another large randomized controlled study (SAMIT trial), which recently completed accrual of 1495 patients in a 2 × 2 design to adjuvant fluoropyrimidine chemotherapy with UFT (uracil/tegafur) or S-1, or sequential paclitaxel and then UFT or S-1, will evaluate the role of taxanes in adjuvant treatment of gastric cancer (see **Table 2**).

Perioperative Chemotherapy

Curative resection (R0) is an important predictor of survival for patients with gastric cancer, and the proportion of patients with R0 resection decreases with increased tumor size and extension.[33] Chemotherapy given before surgery aims to downstage the tumor and increase the chances of a curative resection, thereby leading to improved patient survival. A benefit from perioperative chemotherapy (given before and after surgery) has also been demonstrated in other tumor types such as metastatic colorectal cancer.[34] Preoperative chemotherapy for gastric cancer is generally better tolerated than postoperative treatment, as major surgery (eg, total gastrectomy) can result in long delays before patients are fit enough to start adjuvant treatment, potentially allowing occult micrometastatic disease an opportunity to proliferate. This has been demonstrated by Biffi and colleagues,[35] who directly compared preoperative chemotherapy with the same regimen given postoperatively after gastric surgery. Although this study was closed because of insufficient accrual, increased toxicity and decreased chemotherapy completion rate were observed in the postoperative arm in comparison with the preoperative arm, where the same chemotherapy regimen was given before surgery, thereby reinforcing the challenges involved in giving chemotherapy after gastric surgery.

The most compelling evidence for perioperative chemotherapy comes from the phase 3 United Kingdom Medical Research Adjuvant Gastric Cancer Study[36] (MAGIC), which changed clinical practice across Europe following demonstration of a survival benefit from perioperative chemotherapy. In this trial 503 patients with resectable adenocarcinoma of the stomach, GOJ, or lower esophagus were randomly assigned to either perioperative chemotherapy and surgery or surgery alone. Chemotherapy consisted of 3 preoperative and 3 postoperative cycles of ECF chemotherapy (intravenous epirubicin 50 mg/m^2 and cisplatin 60 mg/m^2 on day 1, and a continuous infusion of 5-fluorouracil 200 mg/m^2 per day for 21 days). The perioperative chemotherapy group demonstrated a significantly improved overall survival (HR 0.75; 95% CI 0.60–0.93; $P = .009$; 5-year survival rate, 36% vs 23%) and progression-free survival (HR 0.66; 95% CI 0.53–0.81; $P<.001$). Patients treated in the chemotherapy arm had a higher rate of curative resections (as deemed by the surgeon; 79.3% vs 70.3%, $P = .03$) and significantly smaller tumors and lower nodal burden than those treated with surgery alone. Preoperative chemotherapy did not increase complications from surgery, and similar rates of postoperative morbidity and 30-day mortality were seen in both arms. No heterogeneity of treatment effect according to the site of primary tumor (stomach, GOJ, or lower esophagus) was demonstrated. This trial also highlighted the challenges involved in delivering postoperative treatment in this patient population group, as 91% of patients who started preoperative chemotherapy completed all 3 cycles of preoperative chemotherapy but only 65% of those who had surgery were able to start postoperative treatment, with only 50% completing all 6 cycles of chemotherapy.

The perioperative approach is also supported by a second phase 3 study, the FNLCC ACCORD 07/FFCD 9703 phase 3 trial,[37] which randomized 224 patients with resectable adenocarcinoma of the stomach, GOJ, or lower esophagus to surgery alone or surgery plus perioperative chemotherapy. Chemotherapy consisted of 2 to 3 preoperative cycles of CF regimen (5-fluorouracil and 800 mg/m^2/d as continuous intravenous infusion days 1–5 and cisplatin 100 mg/m^2 as a 1-hour infusion, every 28 days), and 3 to 4 postoperative cycles of the same regimen in patients who tolerated preoperative treatment well and with no evidence of progressive disease after preoperative chemotherapy, for a total of 6 cycles. The 5-year overall survival was improved by 14% in the chemotherapy arm (38% vs 24%; HR 0.69; 95% CI 0.50–0.95; $P = .02$) compared with the surgery-alone group, and the 5-year DFS was also improved from 21% to 34% with the use of perioperative chemotherapy (HR 0.69; 95% CI 0.50–0.95; $P = .021$). In addition, perioperative chemotherapy significantly improved the rate of curative resection (84% vs 73%; $P = .04$). Although there was increased toxicity in the chemotherapy arm, postoperative morbidity was similar in the two groups. Consistent with the results of the MAGIC[36] study, only 50% of patients could manage to have postoperative chemotherapy compared with nearly 87% who received at least 2 cycles of preoperative chemotherapy, again highlighting the importance of delivering chemotherapy before surgery.

Based on the results of these studies, perioperative chemotherapy with the MAGIC[36] regimen is now widely accepted as a standard treatment across Europe for treating patients with operable, locally advanced adenocarcinoma of the stomach, GOJ, or lower esophagus. Current clinical trials are also using this regimen as a standard to evaluate newer drugs in this setting, although capecitabine has largely replaced infusional 5-fluorouracil, due to the ease of administration and extrapolation from noninferiority data reported in the advanced disease setting.[38] At present there are no data to support a purely neoadjuvant strategy for patients with operable gastric cancer, and patients undergoing preoperative chemotherapy should be treated with postoperative chemotherapy where feasible.

A persistent problem is a relatively low response rate for preoperative chemotherapy, which can occur in up to one-third of patients thus treated. In recent years, response evaluation on positron emission tomography (PET) scan, as measured by a decrease in the tumor glucose standard uptake value (SUV), has been used to predict response to preoperative chemotherapy in patients with tumors of the GOJ.[39] Following treatment with preoperative chemotherapy, early metabolic response in the tumor on the PET scan has been shown to correlate well with the clinical and pathologic response and survival,[40] and perhaps this strategy could potentially help identify patients who fail to respond to preoperative treatment, thereby providing an opportunity to change or intensify their treatment in order to improve treatment outcomes.

NEOADJUVANT STRATEGIES

Neoadjuvant chemotherapy/chemoradiation is commonly used for the operable adenocarcinoma of the esophagus or type I/II GOJ, although as previously stated the perioperative chemotherapy approach is preferred in Europe. The phase 3 United Kingdom OE02[41] study (n = 802), has demonstrated a modest but lasting survival benefit from 2 cycles of neoadjuvant cisplatin and 5-FU given before chemotherapy, with long-term follow-up showing a nearly 6% improvement in overall survival (23% vs 17.1%; P = .03). Neoadjuvant chemoradiation has also been shown to benefit patients with esophageal carcinomas. Walsh and colleagues[42] randomized 113 patients with operable esophageal adenocarcinoma to either 2 cycles of neoadjuvant cisplatin/5-FU chemotherapy with concurrent 40-Gy radiotherapy before surgery, or surgery alone. The median survival was increased from 11 months in the surgery-alone arm to 16 months in the trimodality arm (P = .01). Despite the relatively small sample size and unexpectedly low survival in both arms of the study, trimodality therapy was widely adopted as a treatment strategy in the United States for patients with esophageal adenocarcinomas, though a similar benefit could not be replicated on subsequent studies.[43] A recently reported German study compared neoadjuvant chemotherapy with neoadjuvant chemotherapy followed by chemoradiation in patients with locally advanced GOJ adenocarcinomas.[44] Despite the low accrual this study demonstrated an almost 20% increase in the 3-year survival by the addition of radiotherapy, although the difference was not statistically significant (47.4% vs 27.7%, P = .07), which could potentially be explained by the poor accrual. There was also a statistically insignificant but concerning nearly threefold increase in postoperative mortality from the addition of chemoradiation (10.2% vs 3.8%, P = .26), hence this strategy warrants further evaluation before adoption into routine clinical practice. For patients with esophageal adenocarcinoma histology, benefit has been shown from both neoadjuvant chemotherapy and neoadjuvant chemoradiation in recent meta-analyses,[45,46] although increased pathologic complete response rate and decreased margin positivity were demonstrated from the addition of radiation in a recent randomized trial.[47]

Although the neoadjuvant approach (chemotherapy or chemoradiation) has demonstrated benefit in patients with esophageal adenocarcinoma, there are currently no data to support a purely neoadjuvant approach in patients with gastric cancer. The EORTC 40954 study (n = 144) attempted to answer this question, but the trial was closed because of poor accrual. Although an increased rate of R0 resection was seen (81.9% vs 66.7%, P = .036) with the use of neoadjuvant chemotherapy, no significant benefit in overall survival could be demonstrated (HR 0.84; 95% CI 0.52–1.35; P = .466).[48] Hence this approach should be used only for patients with esophageal or GOJ carcinomas, and patients with stomach cancer should not be treated routinely with this approach. Patients who are treated presurgery with perioperative chemotherapy should be given postoperative treatment where feasible.

SELECTION OF TREATMENT STRATEGY FOR PATIENTS WITH GASTRIC CANCER

All patients with gastric/GOJ adenocarcinomas should be staged with a physical examination and investigations, including full blood count, renal function and liver function blood tests, and endoscopic and computed tomographic scan of the thorax, abdomen, and pelvis (**Fig. 1**). Endoscopic ultrasonography should be performed for tumors of the GOJ to define the T stage and to assess the proximal and distal extent of the disease. Surgery alone can be used to treat patients with early-stage (T1N0) gastric/GOJ adenocarcinoma. For patients with greater than T1N0 operable gastric or type II/III GOJ adenocarcinoma, a laparoscopy should be performed to rule out

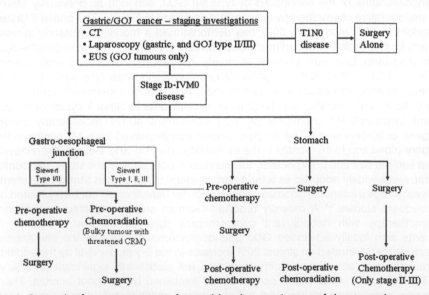

Fig. 1. Strategies for management of operable adenocarcinoma of the stomach or gastroesophageal junction. CRM, circumferential resection margin; CT, computed tomography; EUS, endoscopic ultrasonography; GOJ, gastroesophageal junction.

peritoneal disease. Following this, the authors recommend managing all operable patients (stage Ib–IVa) with a multimodality treatment approach (surgery + chemotherapy ± radiation).

Local expertise is perhaps the single most important factor in how multimodality therapy is used in the management of patients with operable gastric cancer across the world. Whereas adjuvant chemotherapy with S-1 is routinely used after surgery in the Japan, patients in Europe and Australia are managed with a perioperative approach. Patients in the United States have often undergone surgery by the time they are referred to a medical or radiation oncologist, hence the majority are treated with adjuvant chemoradiation. It must be emphasized that all patients should be discussed in a multidisciplinary setting before undergoing surgery. Due to a lack of data for adjuvant chemotherapy in Western patients and high rates of toxicity seen with the postoperative chemoradiation regimen, the authors' recommendation is to use a perioperative chemotherapy approach for managing patients with operable adenocarcinoma of the stomach or GOJ. Also, as preoperative chemotherapy[36,37] leads to a higher rate of curative resections than does surgery alone, adoption of a perioperative approach probably may facilitate a greater proportion of patients with gastric cancer to have a radical procedure.

Management of GOJ carcinomas is an area of controversy, as patients with GOJ carcinomas have been included in the majority of the trials for esophageal as well as gastric carcinomas and hence may be treated using strategies for either operable gastric cancer or esophageal cancer. In general, type I/II GOJ adenocarcinomas are managed as esophagus cancers and type III GOJ adenocarcinomas are managed as gastric cancer. Current data are limited in favoring one approach over the other, and tumor location and local practices may also play a role in selection of the treatment strategy. The authors' preference is to treat GOJ cancers with perioperative chemotherapy, and in general, neoadjuvant chemoradiation is reserved for patients with bulky tumors that are at risk of having an involved circumferential resection margin at the time of surgery. Alternatively, these patients can be treated with neoadjuvant cisplatin/5-FU chemotherapy, and those who do not receive any preoperative treatment may still gain benefit from chemoradiation after surgical resection.

ONGOING TRIALS

Following developments in molecular biology, multiple pathways and targeted agents have now been identified, some of which may be useful in the future treatment of gastric cancer **Table 2**. A notable example is the recognition of the *HER-2* subtype, seen in about 20% to 25% of patients with advanced gastric cancer,[49] although recent data report a much lower rate in East Asia in comparison with the West. In the Japanese ACTS-GC study, the *HER-2* positivity rate was only 13.6%, lower than reports from studies conducted in the Western populations.[50,51] Similarly, in the randomized Korean study of postoperative chemotherapy, the rate of *HER-2* positivity was relatively low, at 8.3%.[52] The phase 3 TOGA study,[53] which preselected patients with advanced gastric cancer for *HER-2* overexpression by immunohistochemistry and fluorescence in situ hybridization, demonstrated a significant improvement in response rate, progression-free survival, and overall survival from the addition of trastuzumab, a monoclonal antibody against *HER-2*, in comparison with cisplatin/5-FU chemotherapy. Given the significant benefit seen in the advanced disease setting, it is possible that a benefit may also be seen from the use of trastuzumab in operable disease. However, this is by no means an easy task because only a small proportion of operable gastric cancer patients will be eligible, therefore conducting a trial that will benefit only a subgroup of patients will require inclusion of a large number of patients and a huge commitment of resources and time. Such studies are most likely to happen in regions with a high prevalence of gastric cancer, such as East Asia, where anti–HER-2 agents could be combined postoperatively with either adjuvant CAPOX or S-1 chemotherapy. For example, even with a very large expected clinical benefit (HR 0.70) of adding trastuzumab to chemotherapy, 400 patients would be required in such a study. With a HER-2 positivity rate of 10% to 15% at best in East Asia, nearly 3000 patients will need to be screened. However, given the current variation in the treatment of operable gastric cancer across the world, results from these trials, even if positive, are unlikely to be applicable elsewhere, therefore trials are needed to evaluate these agents in combination with other strategies as perioperative chemotherapy or adjuvant chemoradiation. Given the additive cardiotoxicity of trastuzumab and anthracyclines, the evaluation of trastuzumab in combination with perioperative ECF chemotherapy is challenging, although a phase 2 Spanish trial is currently evaluating its role with perioperative capecitabine and oxaliplatin chemotherapy without epirubicin. Alternatively, this can be done by combining it with postoperative chemoradiation, but no safety data currently exist to support combining trastuzumab with abdominal chemoradiation.

In the recent phase 3 AVAGAST study,[54] 774 patients with advanced gastric cancer were randomized to cisplatin fluoropyrimidine chemotherapy ± bevacizumab, a monoclonal antibody against vascular endothelial growth factor A. Whereas an overall survival benefit was not observed with the addition of bevacizumab to chemotherapy, a significant improvement was seen in response rate and progression-free survival. In an operable disease setting, a higher response rate to preoperative chemotherapy may translate into a greater rate of R0 resection, and a longer duration of disease control may indeed improve survival from operable gastric cancer. At present, the United Kingdom MRC ST03 study is evaluating the role of bevacizumab in operable gastroesophageal cancer and aims to randomize 950 patients to perioperative ECF chemotherapy ± bevacizumab (see **Table 2**). Early safety data from this study have demonstrated similar rates of toxicity in both arms of the trial.[55]

It is likely that in the coming years we will see multiple other targeted agents that will require evaluation in the treatment of early gastric cancer. However, the current variation in treatment practice will limit wide adoption of any successful strategy/agent across the world. Hence in future, coordination must exist between various gastric cancer trial groups and the pharmaceutical companies to systematically evaluate upcoming novel agents, which is likely to result in wider adoption of a strategy that proves beneficial. This action must also be accompanied with translational research into potential biomarkers as we now begin to realize limitations of the "one size fits all" approach that has generally been used thus far for the management of gastric cancer.

SUMMARY

Despite treatment advances over the past decade, gastric cancer remains one of the most clinically challenging cancers, with generally poor outcomes. Multidisciplinary approach is now accepted as standard for the treatment of operable disease, although marked variation is seen worldwide. In the West, postoperative fluoropyrimidine chemoradiation or perioperative combination chemotherapy is widely used, although a neoadjuvant approach with chemotherapy or chemoradiation may also be used for cancers of the cardia or GOJ. It is hoped that ongoing trials will help identify more efficacious therapies that will permit an individualized approach for the treatment of patients and improve the generally poor prognosis of this aggressive disease.

ACKNOWLEDGMENTS

The authors acknowledge National Health Service funding from the National Institute for Health Research (NIHR) Biomedical Research Center.

REFERENCES

1. Ferlay J, Shin HR, Bray F, et al. 2008, cancer incidence and mortality worldwide: IARC cancerbase no. 10 [internet]. (Lyon France): International Agency for Research on Cancer; 2010. Available at: http://globocan.iarc.fr. Accessed April 26, 2011.
2. Jemal A, Siegel R, Xu J, et al. Cancer statistics, 2010. CA Cancer J Clin 2010; 60(5):277–300.
3. Forman D, Burley VJ. Gastric cancer: global pattern of the disease and an overview of environmental risk factors. Best Pract Res Clin Gastroenterol 2006;20(4): 633–49.
4. Kamangar F, Dores GM, Anderson WF. Patterns of cancer incidence, mortality, and prevalence across five continents: defining priorities to reduce cancer disparities in different geographic regions of the world. J Clin Oncol 2006; 24(14):2137–50.
5. Kubo A, Corley DA. Body mass index and adenocarcinomas of the esophagus or gastric cardia: a systematic review and meta-analysis. Cancer Epidemiol Biomarkers Prev 2006;15(5):872–8.
6. Nakajima T. Gastric cancer treatment guidelines in Japan. Gastric Cancer 2002; 5(1):1–5.
7. Hartgrink HH, van de Velde CJ, Putter H, et al. Extended lymph node dissection for gastric cancer: who may benefit? final results of the randomized Dutch gastric cancer group trial. J Clin Oncol 2004;22(11):2069–77.
8. Cuschieri A, Weeden S, Fielding J, et al. Patient survival after D1 and D2 resections for gastric cancer: long-term results of the MRC randomized surgical trial. Surgical Co-operative Group. Br J Cancer 1999;79(9–10):1522–30.
9. Songun I, Putter H, Kranenbarg EM, et al. Surgical treatment of gastric cancer: 15-year follow-up results of the randomised nationwide Dutch D1D2 trial. Lancet Oncol 2010;11(5):439–49.
10. Hallissey MT, Dunn JA, Ward LC, et al. The second British Stomach Cancer Group trial of adjuvant radiotherapy or chemotherapy in resectable gastric cancer: five-year follow-up. Lancet 1994;343(8909):1309–12.
11. Moertel CG, Childs DS, O'Fallon JR, et al. Combined 5-fluorouracil and radiation therapy as a surgical adjuvant for poor prognosis gastric carcinoma. J Clin Oncol 1984;2(11):1249–54.
12. Gastrointestinal Tumor Study Group. A comparison of combination chemotherapy and combined modality therapy for locally advanced gastric carcinoma. Cancer 1982;49(9):1771–7.
13. Macdonald JS, Smalley SR, Benedetti J, et al. Chemoradiotherapy after surgery compared with surgery alone for adenocarcinoma of the stomach or gastroesophageal junction. N Engl J Med 2001;345(10):725–30.
14. Macdonald JS, Benedetti J, Smalley S, et al. Chemoradiation of resected gastric cancer: a 10-year follow-up of the phase III trial INT0116 (SWOG 9008). J Clin Oncol 2009;27(Suppl):15s [abstract: 4515].
15. Cunningham D, Chua YJ. East meets west in the treatment of gastric cancer. N Engl J Med 2007;357(18):1863–5.
16. Macdonald JS, Smalley S, Benedetti J, et al. Postoperative combined radiation and chemotherapy improves disease-free survival (DFS) and overall survival

(OS) in resected adenocarcinoma of the stomach and gastroesophageal junction: update of the results of Intergroup Study INT-0116 (SWOG 9008). Paper presented at: Gastrointestinal Cancers Symposium. San Francisco, CA, January 22–24, 2004 [abstract: 6].

17. Fuchs CS, Tepper JE, Niedzwiecki D, et al. Postoperative adjuvant chemoradiation for gastric or gastroesophageal junction (GEJ) adenocarcinoma using epirubicin, cisplatin, and infusional (CI) 5-FU (ECF) before and after CI 5-FU and radiotherapy (CRT) compared with bolus 5-FU/LV before and after CRT: intergroup trial CALGB 80101. J Clin Oncol 2011;29(Suppl):[abstract: 4003].

18. Kim S, Lim DH, Lee J, et al. An observational study suggesting clinical benefit for adjuvant postoperative chemoradiation in a population of over 500 cases after gastric resection with D2 nodal dissection for adenocarcinoma of the stomach. Int J Radiat Oncol Biol Phys 2005;63(5):1279–85.

19. Coburn NG, Govindarajan A, Law CH, et al. Stage-specific effect of adjuvant therapy following gastric cancer resection: a population-based analysis of 4,041 patients. Ann Surg Oncol 2008;15(2):500–7.

20. Lee J, Kang W, Lim D, et al. Phase III trial of adjuvant capecitabine/cisplatin (XP) versus capecitabine/cisplatin/RT (XPRT) in resected gastric cancer with D2 nodal dissection (ARTIST trial): safety analysis. J Clin Oncol 2009;27(Suppl):15s [abstract: 4537].

21. Cirera L, Balil A, Batiste-Alentorn E, et al. Randomized clinical trial of adjuvant mitomycin plus tegafur in patients with resected stage III gastric cancer. J Clin Oncol 1999;17(12):3810–5.

22. Neri B, Cini G, Andreoli F, et al. Randomized trial of adjuvant chemotherapy versus control after curative resection for gastric cancer: 5-year follow-up. Br J Cancer 2001;84(7):878–80.

23. Hermans J, Bonenkamp JJ, Boon MC, et al. Adjuvant therapy after curative resection for gastric cancer: meta-analysis of randomized trials. J Clin Oncol 1993;11(8):1441–7.

24. Earle CC, Maroun JA. Adjuvant chemotherapy after curative resection for gastric cancer in non-Asian patients: revisiting a meta-analysis of randomised trials. Eur J Cancer 1999;35(7):1059–64.

25. Mari E, Floriani I, Tinazzi A, et al. Efficacy of adjuvant chemotherapy after curative resection for gastric cancer: a meta-analysis of published randomised trials. A study of the GISCAD (Gruppo Italiano per lo Studio dei Carcinomi dell'Apparato Digerente). Ann Oncol 2000;11(7):837–43.

26. Panzini I, Gianni L, Fattori PP, et al. Adjuvant chemotherapy in gastric cancer: a meta-analysis of randomized trials and a comparison with previous meta-analyses. Tumori 2002;88(1):21–7.

27. Janunger KG, Hafstrom L, Glimelius B. Chemotherapy in gastric cancer: a review and updated meta-analysis. Eur J Surg 2002;168(11):597–608.

28. Sun P, Xiang JB, Chen ZY. Meta-analysis of adjuvant chemotherapy after radical surgery for advanced gastric cancer. Br J Surg 2009;96(1):26–33.

29. Paoletti X, Oba K, Burzykowski T, et al. Benefit of adjuvant chemotherapy for resectable gastric cancer: a meta-analysis. JAMA 2010;303(17):1729–37.

30. Sakuramoto S, Sasako M, Yamaguchi T, et al. Adjuvant chemotherapy for gastric cancer with S-1, an oral fluoropyrimidine. N Engl J Med 2007;357(18):1810–20.

31. Bang Y, Kim Y, Yang H, et al. Adjuvant capecitabine and oxaliplatin for gastric cancer: results of the phase III CLASSIC trial. J Clin Oncol 2011;29(Suppl):[abstract: LBA4002].

32. Sasako M, Kinoshita T, Furukawa H, et al. Five-year results of the randomized phase III trial comparing S-1 monotherapy versus surgery alone for stage II/III gastric cancer patients after curative D2 gastrectomy (ACTS-GC STUDY). Ann Oncol 2010;21(Suppl 8):viii225–49.

33. Siewert JR, Bottcher K, Stein HJ, et al. Relevant prognostic factors in gastric cancer: ten-year results of the German Gastric Cancer Study. Ann Surg 1998; 228(4):449–61.

34. Nordlinger B, Sorbye H, Glimelius B, et al. Perioperative chemotherapy with FOL-FOX4 and surgery versus surgery alone for resectable liver metastases from colorectal cancer (EORTC Intergroup trial 40983): a randomised controlled trial. Lancet 2008;371(9617):1007–16.

35. Biffi R, Fazio N, Luca F, et al. Surgical outcome after docetaxel-based neoadjuvant chemotherapy in locally-advanced gastric cancer. World J Gastroenterol 2010;16(7):868–74.

36. Cunningham D, Allum WH, Stenning SP, et al. Perioperative chemotherapy versus surgery alone for resectable gastroesophageal cancer. N Engl J Med 2006; 355(1):11–20.

37. Ychou M, Boige V, Pignon JP, et al. Perioperative chemotherapy compared with surgery alone for resectable gastroesophageal adenocarcinoma: an FNCLCC and FFCD multicenter phase III trial. J Clin Oncol 2011;29(13): 1715–21.

38. Cunningham D, Starling N, Rao S, et al. Capecitabine and oxaliplatin for advanced esophagogastric cancer. N Engl J Med 2008;358(1):36–46.

39. Lordick F, Ott K, Krause BJ, et al. PET to assess early metabolic response and to guide treatment of adenocarcinoma of the oesophagogastric junction: the MUNI-CON phase II trial. Lancet Oncol 2007;8(9):797–805.

40. Lordick F, Meyer Zum Bueschenfelde C, Herrmann K, et al. PET-guided treatment in locally advanced adenocarcinoma of the esophagogastric junction (AEG): the MUNICON-II study. J Clin Oncol 2011;29(Suppl 4):[abstract: 3].

41. Allum WH, Stenning SP, Bancewicz J, et al. Long-term results of a randomized trial of surgery with or without preoperative chemotherapy in esophageal cancer. J Clin Oncol 2009;27(30):5062–7.

42. Walsh TN, Noonan N, Hollywood D, et al. A comparison of multimodal therapy and surgery for esophageal adenocarcinoma. N Engl J Med 1996;335(7):462–7.

43. Burmeister BH, Smithers BM, Gebski V, et al. Surgery alone versus chemoradiotherapy followed by surgery for resectable cancer of the oesophagus: a randomised controlled phase III trial. Lancet Oncol 2005;6(9):659–68.

44. Stahl M, Walz MK, Stuschke M, et al. Phase III comparison of preoperative chemotherapy compared with chemoradiotherapy in patients with locally advanced adenocarcinoma of the esophagogastric junction. J Clin Oncol 2009; 27(6):851–6.

45. Gebski V, Burmeister B, Smithers BM, et al. Survival benefits from neoadjuvant chemoradiotherapy or chemotherapy in oesophageal carcinoma: a meta-analysis. Lancet Oncol 2007;8(3):226–34.

46. Sjoquist KM, Burmeister BH, Smithers BM, et al. Survival after neoadjuvant chemotherapy or chemoradiotherapy for resectable oesophageal carcinoma: an updated meta-analysis. Lancet Oncol 2011;12:681–92.

47. Burmeister BH, Thomas JM, Burmeister EA, et al. Is concurrent radiation therapy required in patients receiving preoperative chemotherapy for adenocarcinoma of the oesophagus? A randomised phase II trial. Eur J Cancer 2011; 47(3):354–60.

48. Schuhmacher C, Gretschel S, Lordick F, et al. Neoadjuvant chemotherapy compared with surgery alone for locally advanced cancer of the stomach and cardia: European Organisation for Research and Treatment of Cancer randomized trial 40954. J Clin Oncol 2010;28(35):5210–8.

49. Bang Y, Chung H, Xu J, et al. Pathological features of advanced gastric cancer (GC): relationship to human epidermal growth factor receptor 2 (HER2) positivity in the global screening programme of the ToGA trial. J Clin Oncol 2009; 27(Suppl):15s [abstract: 4556].

50. Terashima M, Ochiai A, Kitada K, et al. Impact of human epidermal growth factor receptor (EGFR) and ERBB2 (HER2) expressions on survival in patients with stage II/III gastric cancer, enrolled in the ACTS-GC study. J Clin Oncol 2011; 29(Suppl):[abstract: 4013].

51. Shah MA, Janjigian YY, Pauligk C, et al. Prognostic significance of human epidermal growth factor-2 (HER2) in advanced gastric cancer: a U.S. and European international collaborative analysis. J Clin Oncol 2011;29(Suppl):[abstract: 4014].

52. Park Y, Ryu M, Park H, et al. HER2 status as an independent prognostic marker in patients with advanced gastric cancer receiving adjuvant chemotherapy after curative gastrectomy. J Clin Oncol 2011;29(Suppl):[abstract: 4084].

53. Bang YJ, Van Cutsem E, Feyereislova A, et al. Trastuzumab in combination with chemotherapy versus chemotherapy alone for treatment of HER2-positive advanced gastric or gastro-oesophageal junction cancer (ToGA): a phase 3, open-label, randomised controlled trial. Lancet 2010;376(9742):687–97.

54. Kang Y, Ohtsu A, Van Cutsem E, et al. AVAGAST: a randomized, double-blind, placebo-controlled, phase III study of first-line capecitabine and cisplatin plus bevacizumab or placebo in patients with advanced gastric cancer (AGC). J Clin Oncol 2010;28(Suppl):18s [abstract: LBA4007].

55. Okines AF, Langley RE, Thompson LC, et al. Safety results from a randomized trial of perioperative epirubicin, cisplatin plus capecitabine (ECX) with or without bevacizumab (B) in patients (pts) with gastric or type II/III oesophagogastric junction (OGJ) adenocarcinoma. J Clin Oncol 2011;29(Suppl):[abstract: 4092].

Phase I and II Clinical Trials for Gastric Cancer

Nikhil I. Khushalani, MD

KEYWORDS

• Gastric cancer • Chemotherapy • Targeted agents

Although its global incidence is decreasing, gastric cancer remains a major cause of morbidity and mortality worldwide.[1] It is the second leading cause of cancer-related death worldwide, with the incidence being highest in eastern Asia, eastern Europe, and Latin America. In 2008, it was estimated that nearly 989,600 new cases were diagnosed, with approximately 738,000 deaths from this disease.[2] Most of these cases occur in developing countries. In the United States, approximately 21,500 new cases of gastric cancer will be diagnosed, with 10,500 deaths predicted, in 2011.[3]

Most patients with gastric cancer present at an advanced stage secondary to delayed symptoms. R0 resection remains the only curative modality of treatment. Despite curative attempts at surgery, the 5-year survival remains poor at approximately 20%, with failure patterns including locoregional recurrence and systemic spread. Hence attempts to improve outcomes in this disease have incorporated the use of adjuvant therapy (chemotherapy, radiation therapy, or a combination thereof) or perioperative therapy. These treatment paradigms, including regimens in use, vary across continents. Results from Intergroup 0116 reported in 2001 using adjuvant fluorouracil-based chemoradiotherapy defined the standard of care in the United States.[4] A 10-year follow-up of this trial confirmed the benefit for adjuvant chemoradiation with a hazard ratio of 1.32 for overall survival favoring the treatment arm.[5] The same treatment dogma does not hold true across the Atlantic or the Pacific where perioperative combination chemotherapy or adjuvant treatment with S-1, an oral fluoropyrimidine, is typically recommended based on results of large randomized clinical trials conducted in those continents.[6,7] Notwithstanding the approach used, it has become clear that surgery alone can no longer be recommended as the sole modality of therapy; rather a multimodal treatment plan is appropriate for most patients with localized gastric cancer to optimize the chance for cure.

Disclosures: Research funding for clinical trials: Merck, Pfizer, and National Comprehensive Cancer Network (general research funds from Roche, Allos Therapeutics, and Pfizer).
Roswell Park Cancer Institute, Department of Medicine, Elm and Carlton Streets, Buffalo, NY 14263, USA
E-mail address: nikhil.khushalani@roswellpark.org

Surg Oncol Clin N Am 21 (2012) 113–128
doi:10.1016/j.soc.2011.09.006
1055-3207/12/$ – see front matter © 2012 Elsevier Inc. All rights reserved.

The prognosis in metastatic gastric cancer remains poor and therapy is typically designed for palliation. Systemic chemotherapy improves survival compared with best supportive care and combination chemotherapy yields higher response rates compared with single-agent treatment.[8,9] This treatment is typically recommended for patients with a good performance status. A variety of drugs and combinations are available to choose from, with cisplatin, 5-fluorouracil (5-FU), epirubicin, taxanes, and irinotecan being the most commonly used. Activity of these agents is modest at best and median survival in the advanced setting rarely exceeds 1 year, suggesting that a plateau has been reached in the therapeutic index of available agents in gastric cancer. Hence there is an urgent need to identify novel drugs. Improved understanding of the biology of neoplasia has allowed definition of cellular pathways that result in the growth, replication, and inhibition of apoptosis in the cancer cell. The focus of research efforts has now moved from examining traditional cytotoxic chemotherapy to evaluating biologic compounds that specifically target the tumor or its microenvironment. There is ample evidence that molecular markers in gastric cancer may provide prognostic data in addition to clinical staging. Some markers studied to date include DNA copy number, microsatellite instability, thymidylate synthase (TS), E-cadherin, β-catenin, p53, cyclooxygenase-2 (COX-2), vascular endothelial growth factor receptor (VEGFR), epidermal growth factor receptor (EGFR), and matrix metalloproteinases (MMPs).[10] Development of drugs that target some of these receptors and proteases may lead to a higher therapeutic gain. Early phase clinical trials examining this is the focus of this review after an initial discussion on the commonly used chemotherapy regimens.

CHEMOTHERAPY IN ADVANCED GASTRIC CANCER

A standard regimen in advanced gastric cancer (AGC) remains an enigma because large, randomized clinical trials conducted in the past 3 decades have failed to establish a single regimen as being superior to others. Important considerations for individualized treatment include performance status, nutritional status, and comorbidities. It is common for patients with esophagogastric cancer to present with varying degrees of caloric malnutrition secondary to mechanical obstruction, impaired gastric motility, early satiety, and anorexia. In the meta-analysis by Wagner and colleagues,[8] triplet drug therapy containing 5-FU, cisplatin, and an anthracycline resulted in the best overall survival. The regimen of epirubicin, cisplatin, and infusion 5-FU (ECF) has been commonly used in Europe in the first-line setting.[11,12] In the Randomized ECF for Advanced and Locally Advanced Esophagogastric Cancer 2 (REAL-2) trial, the combination of epirubicin, oxaliplatin, and capecitabine (EOX) was determined to be as effective as ECF in therapy-naïve patients, and had a more favorable toxicity profile.[13] The response rate to EOX was 47% and the median survival was 11.2 months. This trial clearly showed that oxaliplatin and capecitabine could safely be substituted for cisplatin and 5-FU respectively without compromise of efficacy. This finding also mitigates the need for central venous access. In the V325 study, the triple-drug combination of docetaxel, cisplatin, and 5-FU (DCF) was superior to cisplatin plus 5-FU, although at the risk of considerable toxicity.[14] The high rate of toxicity (complicated neutropenia, 29%; diarrhea, 19%) with this regimen has tempered enthusiasm for its use in the palliative setting and modifications to the doses and schedules of the drugs have been investigated. A modified DCF (mDCF) regimen with dose attenuations in cisplatin and docetaxel along with a shortened infusion 5-FU schedule was tested in a multicenter phase II trial with an impressive response rate of 52% in the 41 evaluable patients assigned to the mDCF arm.[15] The 6-month progression-free survival (PFS) was 57% (95% confidence interval [CI], 37–73) and the median overall survival (OS) was 15.1 months (95% CI, 9–25). Other regimens that are frequently used include irinotecan in combination with cisplatin or leucovorin-modulated 5-FU (FOLFIRI).[16,17] Combinations of oxaliplatin plus a fluoropyrimidine are well tolerated and consistently elicit response rates of 40% to 50% in metastatic gastric cancer.[16,18–20]

In the absence of direct comparison studies, it is not clear whether the triplet combinations mentioned earlier are necessarily superior to doublet therapy when the more modern drugs including oxaliplatin, irinotecan, taxanes, capecitabine, and S-1 are used. The literature is replete with numerous phase II trials exploring different doses, schedules, and combinations of these drugs, but breaking the 1 year median survival in metastatic gastric cancer using chemotherapy has proved an elusive goal. In 2010, the ToGA (Transtuzumab for Gastric Cancer) trial reported positive results for the addition of transtuzumab to a standard platinum-fluoropyrimidine doublet in patients with Her2-positive gastric and gastroesophageal junction cancer, achieving a median survival of 13.8 months (95% CI, 12–17).[21] This is discussed in more detail later. A brief summary of commonly used regimens in the front-line setting is provided in **Table 1**. Although this is not an exhaustive list, it summarizes the options that are available, the need for individualizing therapy, and it underscores the need to build on them using chemotherapy as a backbone. Thus far, the heterogeneity of gastric cancers has not allowed for the identification of a dominant driver mutation that is amenable to drug therapy'.[22]

INHIBITORS OF ANGIOGENESIS

Angiogenesis, the process of formation of new blood vessels from existing vasculature, is fundamental to normal physiologic development and also to the development of tumors and the phenomenon of metastasis.[23–25] The vascular endothelial growth factor (VEGF) family and its receptors are key mediators in angiogenesis and have been exploited as targets for therapeutic intervention. Numerous factors stimulate and regulate the VEGF/VEGFR axis, important among them being hypoxia.[26] In addition, crosstalk with other molecular pathways adds to the complexity of this mechanism of tumorigenesis, as shown by upregulation of VEGF and neuropilin-1 expression in gastric cancer cell lines by activation of the EGFR pathway.[27] Increased serum or tumor VEGF levels have been found to correlate with nodal metastases, liver

Table 1
Commonly used front-line chemotherapy regimens in AGC

Regimens	Phase	Number of Patients	Response Rate (%)	OS (mo)
ECF/EOX[13]	3	1002	41, 48	9.9, 11.2
DCF[14]	3	445	37	9.2
mDCF[15]	2	72	52	15.1
Cisplatin+capecitabine[99]	3	316	46	10.5
Cisplatin/irinotecan[16]	2	38	58	9.0
FOLFIRI[17]	2	136	40	11.3
FOLFOX[19]	2	61	38	11.2

Abbreviation: FOLFOX, oxaliplatin plus leucovorin-modulated 5-FU.

metastases, and poor prognosis in gastric cancer.[28–32] Strategies for interruption of this pathway include ligand and receptor tyrosine kinase blockade.

Monoclonal Antibodies

Bevacizumab, an anti-VEGF-A humanized monoclonal antibody, is currently approved in the United States for the treatment of colorectal cancer, lung cancer, kidney cancer, and recurrent glioblastoma. Following encouraging results from the addition of bevacizumab to chemotherapy in colorectal cancer, its evaluation in other tumors of the gastrointestinal tract was a natural and rationale succession plan. Shah and colleagues[33] from the Memorial Sloan Kettering Cancer Institute reported an impressive 65% response rate in a phase II trial of 42 patients with advanced gastric or gastroesophageal junction (GEJ) carcinoma from the addition of bevacizumab administered on day 1 to combination cisplatin and irinotecan given on days 1 and 8 in a 21-day cycle of therapy. The median time to progression was 8.3 months (95% CI, 5.5–9.9 months) and median OS was 12.3 months (95% CI, 11.3–17.2 months). One-fourth of the patients experienced a grade 3 or 4 thromboembolic event and 28% developed grade 3 hypertension, both now well-known adverse effects of this drug. Three additional phase II trials have examined the addition of bevacizumab to different chemotherapeutic regimens reporting response rates of 42% to 67%.[34–36] In the study of bevacizumab plus mDCF, the 6-month PFS was 79%, median PFS was 12 months (95% CI, 8.8–18.2 months), and median OS was 16.8 months (95% CI, 12.1–26.1 months).[36] Patients with the diffuse variant of gastric cancer had poorer outcomes compared with proximal and GEJ tumors. Thirty-nine percent of patients developed a grade 3 or 4 thromboembolic event, although more than half of these patients were asymptomatic. This high rate of thrombotic events and the need for therapeutic anticoagulation warrant caution in the ongoing study of bevacizumab in this setting.

The AVAGAST (Avastin in Gastric Cancer) trial was an international effort that followed the phase II trials mentioned earlier to better define the role of bevacizumab in the treatment of gastric cancer.[37] Of 917 eligible patients with locally advanced unresectable or metastatic gastric or GEJ cancer, 774 were randomized to receive a cisplatin-fluoropyrimidine (capecitabine or infusion 5-FU) doublet with or without bevacizumab administered every 21 days. The statistical plan hypothesized that the addition of the biologic agent would improve the median OS from 10 months to 12.8 months. Bevacizumab improved response rates (46% vs 37.4%, $P = .0315$) and median PFS (6.7 months vs 5.3 months; hazard ratio, 0.80; $P = .037$) but failed to significantly affect OS (12.1 months with bevacizumab plus chemotherapy vs 10.1 months for placebo plus chemotherapy, $P = .1002$; hazard ratio, 0.87; 95% CI, 0.73–1.03). The addition of bevacizumab did not seem to cause an increase in clinically significant toxicity apart from diarrhea and the hand-foot syndrome. The rate of thromboembolic events was more common in the placebo arm (9%) compared with the bevacizumab group (6%). The remainder toxicity profile was commensurate with what is known for this agent. Although these negative results will likely inhibit further development of bevacizumab in the treatment of gastric cancer, some interesting observations from these trials may suggest that certain populations of patients may benefit and need further study. Second-line chemotherapy was more frequently administered in the Pan-Asian population (66%) within this study cohort compared with the Pan-European (31%) and Pan-American (21%) counterparts. Patients treated in the Pan-American cohort seemed to derive benefit from the addition of bevacizumab to chemotherapy (median OS, 11.5 months vs 6.8 months for placebo; hazard ratio, 0.63; 95% CI, 0.43–0.93) compared with the Pan-Asian subgroup. This adds further credibility to the notion that there may be inherent biologic differences in gastric cancer behavior based on geographic regions of the world. The dose of bevacizumab used in AVAGAST was lower (7.5 mg/kg every 21 days) compared with the trials mentioned earlier that used 10 or 15 mg/kg every 21 days. Pooling data (n = 156) from 5 US investigator-initiated clinical trials using bevacizumab plus chemotherapy in AGC, Smyth and colleagues[38] attempted to contrast the Western experience with the population treated on the AVAGAST trial. Significant differences were noted in the location of the primary tumor (GEJ more frequent in the United States), histology (diffuse histology less common in the United States), and presence of liver metastases (more common in the US cohort). The median OS for the diffuse gastric cancer, non-diffuse gastric cancer, and GEJ cancer was 12 months, 15 months, and 20 months respectively (P = .02), with pooled OS of 14 months (95% CI, 12–16 months) Hence further investigation of this antibody in combination with chemotherapy in AGC learning from lessons derived from these early, hypothesis-generating trials is warranted.

All the trials listed earlier discontinued bevacizumab on progression of disease. Little is known about continuation of this agent with second-line chemotherapy or its use as part of a second-line regimen after failure of chemotherapy alone. Early stage clinical trials to this effect are ongoing. Similarly, bevacizumab is also being investigated in the context of multimodal therapy for localized gastric cancer but efficacy data are not yet available. Early reports have outlined its safety in this setting without any significant increase in the risk of perioperative complications.[35,39,40]

Another antiangiogenic antibody that has shown promise in early study is ramucirumab. It is a fully human immunoglobulin G1 monoclonal antibody that targets the extracellular domain of VEGFR-2 with high affinity. Preclinical studies showed efficacy in several tumor types.[41] In a phase I dose-finding study, 37 patients with solid tumors refractory to standard therapy were treated with weekly ramucirumab in doses ranging from 2 mg/kg to 16 mg/kg.[42] Dose-limiting toxicities included hypertension, venous thrombosis, proteinuria, and vomiting. In patients with measurable disease, the response rate was 15%. One patient with gastric cancer (dose 4 mg/kg) experienced a partial response that lasted for 103 weeks. Secondary end points in this trial included pharmacodynamic marker sampling (VEGF-A, sVEGFR-1, sVEGFR-2) and measurement of perfusion and vascularity in liver metastases by dynamic contrast-enhanced magnetic resonance imaging (DCE-MRI). Clinical trials of ramucirumab as a single agent or in combination with paclitaxel in advanced gastric, esophageal, and GEJ cancers are currently underway.

Receptor Tyrosine Kinase Inhibitors

Unlike the monoclonal antibodies, the numerous antiangiogenic receptor tyrosine kinase inhibitors (TKI) in clinical development have multiple targets. Some of these agents include sunitinib, axitinib, pazopanib, sorafenib, and vandetanib. However, they have limited activity as single agents in gastric cancer. In 2 phase II trials, sunitinib as monotherapy after failure of first-line therapy in AGC elicited response rates of less than 5%.[43,44] In both trials, the US Food and Drug Administration (FDA)–approved dosing schedule of 50 mg daily for 4 weeks followed by a break for 2 weeks was adopted. The toxicities conformed to its known profile and included myelosuppression, nausea, fatigue, anorexia, diarrhea, and stomatitis. With its limited single-agent activity, further investigation of this agent would have to involve a backbone of chemotherapy. At our institution, we are conducting a phase I trial of sunitinib added to irinotecan and leucovorin-modulated infusion 5-FU (FOLFIRI) in therapy-naïve patients with advanced gastric or GEJ carcinoma.[45] Our initial experience led to alterations in sunitinib dosing to an intermittent schedule of 14 days in a 28-day cycle along with dose attenuation of biweekly FOLFIRI. A standard 3-plus-3 phase I design is being used with the sunitinib dose starting at 25 mg/d with escalations in increments of 12.5 mg. Pharmacokinetic parameters for sunitinib, irinotecan, and SN-38 are being measured. Accrual to this trial is currently ongoing.

The RAS-mitogen–activated protein kinase (MAPK) pathway plays a central role in regulating cellular signaling, growth, and survival.[46] *Raf* is an essential serine-threonine kinase that functions as an effector downstream of *Ras*.[47] The MAPK pathway has been shown to upregulate VEGF expression through hypoxia-inducible factor-1α.[48] Sorafenib is a multitargeted TKI that inhibits activation of the MAPK pathway (by abrogating the activity of *c-raf* and *b-raf*) and extracellular signal-regulated kinase (ERK) phosphorylation. In addition, it is a potent inhibitor of VEGFR-2 and VEGFR-3, platelet-derived growth factor receptor, Flt-3, c-kit, and fibroblast growth factor receptor-1. Sorafenib has regulatory approval in the United States for the treatment of hepatocellular carcinoma and renal cell carcinoma. In gastric cancer xenografts, sorafenib inhibited cellular proliferation and angiogenesis.[48] In a phase I clinical trial in gastric cancer, sorafenib was combined with capecitabine and cisplatin, achieving a response rate of 63% and an OS of 14.7 months (95% CI, 12–20 months).[49] The dose-limiting toxicities of this combination were diarrhea and neutropenia; sorafenib at 400 mg twice daily, with capecitabine 800 mg/m^2 twice daily on days 1 to 14, and cisplatin 60 mg/m^2 on day 1 of a 21-day cycle, was the recommended dose for further study. In the Eastern Cooperative Oncology Group (ECOG) Trial 5203, sorafenib was added to docetaxel and cisplatin in therapy-naïve patients with gastric or GEJ cancer (n = 44).[50] Eighteen of 44 patients attained a partial response (41%) with a median PFS of 5.8 months and median OS of 13.6 months. The principle toxicity was neutropenia (grades 3 and 4), seen in two-thirds of the patients treated. There were 2 treatment-related deaths in this cohort.

Other TKIs are undergoing study in AGC, including phase I evaluation of cediranib with cisplatin plus a fluoropyrimidine and phase II study of pazopanib in combination with capecitaine and oxaliplatin. Results from these trials are forthcoming.

Based on reported data, it is unlikely that the addition of antiangiogenic receptor TKIs will dramatically alter the therapeutic landscape in gastric cancer. Biomarker and pharmacodynamic end points must be mandated in future studies to establish whether there is a cohort of patients with this disease that would benefit from their addition.

STRATEGIES TARGETING THE EGFR

The epidermal growth factor receptors are transmembrane glycoprotein tyrosine kinases that are critical for tumor cell proliferation, invasion, and metastases.[51] Overexpression of EGFR detected by immunohistochemistry is common in gastroesophageal cancer, making it a natural target for therapeutic intervention.[52–54] This overexpression has been linked to poorer prognosis in gastric cancer.[55] Similar to antiangiogenic therapy, both ligand interference and tyrosine kinase blockade are methods of interrupting cascade signaling via this pathway; these avenues have been successfully exploited in colorectal, pancreatic, lung, and head and neck cancers.

Cetuximab is a chimeric monoclonal antibody that targets the extracellular domain of EGFR, resulting in competitive inhibition of ligand binding, abrogation of tyrosine kinase activity, and eventual receptor downregulation. In colorectal cancer, the presence of *k-ras* mutations is predictive for nonresponse to cetuximab.[56] The frequency of these mutations in gastroesophageal cancers is probably far less.[57] Cetuximab has been extensively studied in gastric cancer as monotherapy, in combination with other agents, and in the locally advanced setting. In a phase II trial, Chan and colleagues[58] evaluated the single-agent activity of cetuximab in metastatic gastric and esophagus cancer following failure of 1 or 2 prior regimens of therapy. Although treatment was well tolerated with known effects such as acneiform rash, fatigue, diarrhea, and hypomagnesemia, the response rate was only 3% and the stable disease rate was 6% among 30 evaluable patients. A similar efficacy has been reported in esophageal cancer in the Southwest Oncology Group (SWOG) Trial 0415, which failed to meet its primary end point achieving a 6-month survival of 36% (95% CI, 24%, 50%).[59] Although these results suggest minimal activity of cetuximab as a single agent, there is a preclinical rationale for its synergistic combination with chemotherapy in gastric cancer through downregulation of the EGFR pathway.[60] It has been explored with several chemotherapy doublets including platinums, fluoropyrimidines, irinotecan, and docetaxel.[61–63] In these trials, the response rate has ranged from 41% to 65% and, inherent to selection bias in the phase II setting, impressive median survivals were also noted. In the German Arbeitsgemeinschaft Internistische Onkologie (AIO), patients with AGC or GEJ cancer received 6-weekly doses of cetuximab (after an initial loading dose), irinotecan, and infusion 5-FU in a 50-day cycle as first-line therapy.[64] The disease control rate was 79%, PFS was 9.0 months (95% CI, 7.1, 15.6) and median OS was 16.5 months (95% CI, 11.7, 30.1). Disease response was more commonly seen in EGFR-expressing tumors ($P = .041$). There was no relation of response or survival to the development of skin rash. The investigators acknowledged the limitations associated with their small sample size. The most promising regimens for further study with cetuximab include fluoropyrimidines with oxaliplatin or irinotecan, and phase III evaluations are underway. However, results from predictive and/or prognostic markers in these studies have been inconsistent and are too preliminary for conclusive interpretation.

Matuzumab, a humanized anti-EGFR monoclonal antibody, was evaluated by Rao and colleagues[65,66] in separate phase I and randomized phase II trials in combination with the epirubicin, cisplatin, capecitabine (ECX) chemotherapy regimen. However, it did not add to the efficacy of chemotherapy and further study of this drug in gastric cancer has been largely abandoned. Panitumumab is another humanized monoclonal antibody approved for use in metastatic colorectal cancer. It is being examined in the REAL-3 study in Europe in the first-line setting with a plan to randomize 730 patients to EOX with or without panitumumab following the reporting of the initial safety data with this combination that necessitated dose modifications to the EOX regimen.[67]

Erlotinib and gefitinib are small-molecule TKIs targeting the EGFR pathway. Phase II trials have shown modest efficacy as single agents in AGC. In SWOG 0127, a phase II, open-labeled, multicenter trial, 68 eligible therapy-naïve patients (43 GEJ, 25 gastric) were treated with erlotinib at a dose of 150 mg daily.[53] There were no objective responses seen in the gastric cancer cohort and accrual to this group was discontinued. Four responses (9%, 95% CI, 3, 22) were seen in the GEJ stratum. OS for the GEJ and gastric cancer cohorts was 6.7 months and 3.5 months respectively. There were no mutations identified in exons 18, 19, or 21 of the *EGFR* gene within available tumor tissue samples (n = 54), nor was there evidence of EGFR amplification in tested samples from responders. The differential responses between the GEJ and gastric cancer cohorts in this study, albeit small, add further credibility to the theory that cancers arising in these anatomic regions are different at a molecular level, leading to differences in biologic behavior and sensitivity to therapy.

Targeting Her2 (erb2)

Her2 is a member of the EGFR family, which initiates cascade signaling after undergoing homodimerization or heterodimerization with other members of this family.[68] Its function and therapeutic targeting has been studied exhaustively in breast cancer. In gastric cancer, overexpression or amplification of Her2 is seen and may be associated with a poorer prognosis, though data are conflicting.[69–71] Transtuzumab is a humanized monoclonal antibody directed against the Her2 receptor and is standard of care in the treatment of Her2-expressing breast cancer, both in the metastatic and adjuvant settings. In gastric cancer xenograft models, transtuzumab showed efficacy as monotherapy and also enhanced the activity of several chemotherapeutic agents including cisplatin, paclitaxel, irinotecan, and capecitabine.[72] In the international ToGA trial, 810 of 3665 (22%) successfully screened patients of advanced gastric or GEJ cancer were Her2 positive, of whom 594 were randomized to receive cisplatin plus a fluoropyrimidine (capecitabine, 5-FU) with or without transtuzumab.[21] Crossover to transtuzumab was not permitted at the time of disease progression. Transtuzumab improved the response rate (47% vs 35%, $P = .0017$), PFS (6.7 months vs 5.5 months, $P = .0004$), and OS (13.8 months vs 11.1 months; hazard ratio 0.74; 95% CI, 0.60, 0.91; $P = .0046$). There was no increase in cardiotoxicity in the experimental arm of this study. These results led to the regulatory approval of transtuzumab in the United States in October 2010 for Her2-positive metastatic gastric and GEJ carcinoma in combination with chemotherapy in the front-line setting. It is hoped that this successful large trial will serve as an impetus to develop more selection-driven studies in gastroesophageal cancers that use a molecular classification of patients and their tumors. Although a trial examining transtuzumab in the adjuvant setting may seem an obvious continuum in this field, several questions arise. The small percentage of Her2-positive gastric cancer, especially in a Western population, suggests that a large trial needs to be designed if a significant difference effect is to be shown. In addition, the intestinal variant of gastric cancer is more likely to be Her2 positive compared with the diffuse subtype, the latter being more commonly seen in the West, as was confirmed in an international collaboration effort with results being reported recently.[73] In addition, the potential for cardiotoxicity related to transtuzumab in the perioperative setting, with an anthracycline (eg, as part of the EOX regimen), or in the context of postoperative radiotherapy (common in the United States) need to be considerations in this investigation.

As shown in the ToGA trial, both primary and secondary resistance to transtuzumab is inevitable. A potential strategy to overcome this by developing a transtuzumab-DM1 conjugate has been explored in breast cancer.[74] DM1, a derivative of maytansine-1, is a cytotoxic molecule that inhibits microtubule assembly. The conjugate delivers this molecule to Her2-expressing cells via receptor-mediated endocytosis and the active moiety is released by lysosomal degradation. This approach has been tested in preclinical models of Her2-expressing gastric cancer with promising antitumor effect, thereby warranting further exploration in the clinical setting.[75]

Lapatinib is an oral small-molecule TKI that is a dual inhibitor of EGFR and Her2. In SWOG 0413, a response rate of 9% and OS of 4.8 months were observed in 47 unselected patients with gastric cancers treated with lapatinib dosed at 1500 mg daily.[76] Grade 4 toxicities reported included myocardial ischemia, fatigue, and emesis. Further development of lapatinib in gastric cancer will involve combinations with chemotherapy or other targeted agents that have sound preclinical rationales.[77,78]

MAMMALIAN TARGET OF RAPAMYCIN AND ITS INHIBITION

The mammalian target of rapamycin (mTOR), activated by the PI3 kinase pathway, is a critical protein kinase involved in the regulation of cellular growth and cell cycle progression.[79] Dysregulation of the mTOR pathway has been described in gastric cancer and may be prognostic.[80,81] Everolimus is an oral rapamycin derivative that inhibits mTOR and downstream phosphorylation, eventually resulting in cell cycle arrest. Responses in gastric and esophageal cancer were noted in a phase I study of everolimus in refractory solid tumors in Japan.[82] In a phase II trial (n = 53) in treated gastric cancer (≤2 prior regimens), no responses were seen. The disease control rate was 56% (95% CI, 41.3, 70), median PFS was 2.7 months (95% CI, 1.6, 3), and median OS was 10.1 months (95% CI, 6.5, 12.1).[83] Common toxicities observed included anemia, lymphopenia, and hyponatremia. Grade 1 and 2 pneumonitis occurred in 15% of patients. There was no difference in efficacy based on the number of prior treatment regimens. The high disease control rate has prompted additional trials of this drug that are ongoing. In a phase I trial of everolimus and capecitabine in heavily pretreated gastric cancer conducted in Korea, everolimus at 5 mg twice daily uninterrupted combined with capecitabine at 650 mg/m^2 twice daily for 14 days every 21 days was determined to be the recommended dose for further study.[84] The toxicity profile was tolerable and a phase II trial of this combination is underway.

OTHER NOVEL APPROACHES TO THERAPY IN GASTRIC CANCER
Mesenchymal-Epithelial Transition Factor

The hepatocyte growth factor (HGF) is the physiologic ligand for the receptor tyrosine kinase mesenchymal-epithelial transition factor (c-MET). Signaling through this pathway activates numerous downstream effectors including PI3K/Akt, Ras/Raf/MEK/ERK, and focal adhesion kinase (FAK) pathways and plays an important role in cancer cell survival[85,86] Activation of c-MET secondary to mutations or MET amplification may be important in gastric cancer tumorigenesis, although this may be rare in the Western population.[87–89] In a phase I trial of ARQ-197, an oral, selective c-MET inhibitor, 1 patient with AGC had stable disease lasting for 15 weeks.[90] A minor regression in the size of hepatic metastasis was noted in this patient. The most frequent adverse events were fatigue, nausea, and vomiting. Foretinib is a dual c-MET and VEGFR-2 inhibitor that is undergoing testing in early stage clinical trials including gastric cancer.[91,92] Pharmacodynamic end points are being studied to better understand target inhibition of this pathway.

Histone Deacetylase Inhibitors

Transforming growth factor β (TGF-β) is thought to play an important role in the growth inhibition of normal epithelium and many cancer types, including gastric cancer.[93] TGF-β functions through 2 cell surface receptors, type I (RI) and type II (RII). Vorinostat, an oral histone deacetylase (HDAC) inhibitor approved in cutaneous T-cell lymphoma, has been shown to induce RI and restore TGF-β response.[94] Using this observation, we hypothesized that HDAC inhibition by vorinostat may augment response to chemotherapy in advanced gastric and esophageal cancers. We have completed accrual to a phase I study of vorinostat with FOLFIRI evaluating continuous and intermittent oral dosing of the former drug.[95] Secondary end points include examination of survivin and TGF-β expression. The major toxicities encountered have been myelosuppression, fatigue, and diarrhea.

Table 2 Molecular targets in gastric cancer		
VEGFR	HDAC	COX-2
EGFR	CDK	Heat shock protein
Her2	Proteasome	
mTOR	IGF-1R	
c-MET	Matrix metalloproteinase	

Cell Cycle Inhibitors

Cyclin-dependent kinases (CDK) are regulators of the cell cycle that ensure orderly progression of this cellular function. Flavopiridol is a pan-CDK inhibitor that has been evaluated in gastric cancer as a single agent in a phase II trial.[96] There were no objective responses and higher incidences of vascular thromboses and fatigue were noted. Further study of this drug has been in combination with chemotherapy including irinotecan and the taxanes.[97]

Others

There are several other novel compounds that are in early stages of investigation in gastric cancer. Those that seem promising include proteasome inhibitors (bortezomib) and inhibitors of the type-1 insulinlike growth factor receptor (IGF-1R). Mature results from these trials are awaited. A list of the common therapeutic targets in this disease is given in **Table 2**.

SUMMARY

Gastric cancer remains a global public health problem with considerable heterogeneity in pathogenesis and clinical presentation across geographic regions. Improved understanding of the molecular biology of this disease has opened avenues for targeted intervention.[98] It is becoming increasingly clear that an individualized treatment approach is required for optimal management of this cancer. Strategies to overcoming resistance to therapy include combining targeted agents with the traditional options of chemotherapy/radiation therapy, and also targeting more than 1 pathway of carcinogenesis at a time. Encouraging molecular hypothesis and biomarker-driven trials will lead to improved patient outcomes and may eventually enable the therapeutic nihilism associated with gastric cancer to be overcome.

REFERENCES

1. Bertuccio P, Chatenoud L, Levi F, et al. Recent patterns in gastric cancer: a global overview. Int J Cancer 2009;125(3):666–73.
2. Jemal A, Bray F, Center MM, et al. Global cancer statistics. CA Cancer J Clin 2011;61(2):69–90.
3. Siegel R, Ward E, Brawley O, et al. Cancer statistics, 2011: the impact of eliminating socioeconomic and racial disparities on premature cancer deaths. CA Cancer J Clin 2011;61(4):212–36.
4. Macdonald JS, Smalley SR, Benedetti J, et al. Chemoradiotherapy after surgery compared with surgery alone for adenocarcinoma of the stomach or gastroesophageal junction. N Engl J Med 2001;345(10):725–30.

5. Macdonald JS, Benedetti J, Smalley S, et al. Chemoradiation of resected gastric cancer: A 10-year follow-up of the phase III trial INT0116 (SWOG 9008). ASCO Meeting Abstracts. Orlando (FL), June 8, 2009;27(15S):4515.
6. Cunningham D, Allum WH, Stenning SP, et al. Perioperative chemotherapy versus surgery alone for resectable gastroesophageal cancer. N Engl J Med 2006; 355(1):11–20.
7. Sakuramoto S, Sasako M, Yamaguchi T, et al. Adjuvant chemotherapy for gastric cancer with S-1, an oral fluoropyrimidine. N Engl J Med 2007;357(18):1810–20.
8. Wagner AD, Grothe W, Haerting J, et al. Chemotherapy in advanced gastric cancer: a systematic review and meta-analysis based on aggregate data. J Clin Oncol 2006;24(18):2903–9.
9. Rivera F, Vega-Villegas ME, Lopez-Brea MF. Chemotherapy of advanced gastric cancer. Cancer Treat Rev 2007;33(4):315–24.
10. Scartozzi M, Galizia E, Freddari F, et al. Molecular biology of sporadic gastric cancer: prognostic indicators and novel therapeutic approaches. Cancer Treat Rev 2004;30(5):451–9.
11. Findlay M, Cunningham D, Norman A, et al. A phase II study in advanced gastro-esophageal cancer using epirubicin and cisplatin in combination with continuous infusion 5-fluorouracil (ECF). Ann Oncol 1994;5(7):609–16.
12. Zaniboni A, Barni S, Labianca R, et al. Epirubicin, cisplatin, and continuous infusion 5-fluorouracil is an active and safe regimen for patients with advanced gastric cancer. An Italian Group for the Study of Digestive Tract Cancer (GISCAD) report. Cancer 1995;76(10):1694–9.
13. Cunningham D, Starling N, Rao S, et al. Capecitabine and oxaliplatin for advanced esophagogastric cancer. N Engl J Med 2008;358(1):36–46.
14. Van Cutsem E, Moiseyenko VM, Tjulandin S, et al. Phase III study of docetaxel and cisplatin plus fluorouracil compared with cisplatin and fluorouracil as first-line therapy for advanced gastric cancer: a report of the V325 Study Group. J Clin Oncol 2006;24(31):4991–7.
15. Shah MA, Shibata S, Stoller RG, et al. Random assignment multicenter phase II study of modified docetaxel, cisplatin, fluorouracil (mDCF) versus DCF with growth factor support (GCSF) in metastatic gastroesophageal adenocarcinoma (GE). ASCO Meeting Abstracts. Orlando (FL), June 14, 2010;28(Suppl 15):4014.
16. Ajani JA, Baker J, Pisters PW, et al. CPT-11 plus cisplatin in patients with advanced, untreated gastric or gastroesophageal junction carcinoma: results of a phase II study. Cancer 2002;94(3):641–6.
17. Bouche O, Raoul JL, Bonnetain F, et al. Randomized multicenter phase II trial of a biweekly regimen of fluorouracil and leucovorin (LV5FU2), LV5FU2 plus cisplatin, or LV5FU2 plus irinotecan in patients with previously untreated metastatic gastric cancer: a Federation Francophone de Cancerologie Digestive Group Study–FFCD 9803. J Clin Oncol 2004;22(21):4319–28.
18. Al-Batran SE, Atmaca A, Hegewisch-Becker S, et al. Phase II trial of biweekly infusional fluorouracil, folinic acid, and oxaliplatin in patients with advanced gastric cancer. J Clin Oncol 2004;22(4):658–63.
19. De Vita F, Orditura M, Matano E, et al. A phase II study of biweekly oxaliplatin plus infusional 5-fluorouracil and folinic acid (FOLFOX-4) as first-line treatment of advanced gastric cancer patients. Br J Cancer 2005;92(9):1644–9.
20. Jatoi A, Murphy BR, Foster NR, et al. Oxaliplatin and capecitabine in patients with metastatic adenocarcinoma of the esophagus, gastroesophageal junction and gastric cardia: a phase II study from the North Central Cancer Treatment Group. Ann Oncol 2006;17(1):29–34.

21. Bang YJ, Van Cutsem E, Feyereislova A, et al. Trastuzumab in combination with chemotherapy versus chemotherapy alone for treatment of HER2-positive advanced gastric or gastro-oesophageal junction cancer (ToGA): a phase 3, open-label, randomised controlled trial. Lancet 2010;376(9742):687–97.
22. Owens J. Determining druggability. Nat Rev Drug Discov 2007;6(3):187.
23. Folkman J. What is the evidence that tumors are angiogenesis dependent? J Natl Cancer Inst 1990;82(1):4–6.
24. Ferrara N. Vascular endothelial growth factor as a target for anticancer therapy. Oncologist 2004;9(Suppl 1):2–10.
25. Carmeliet P. Angiogenesis in health and disease. Nat Med 2003;9(6):653–60.
26. Ferrara N, Gerber HP, LeCouter J. The biology of VEGF and its receptors. Nat Med 2003;9(6):669–76.
27. Akagi M, Kawaguchi M, Liu W, et al. Induction of neuropilin-1 and vascular endothelial growth factor by epidermal growth factor in human gastric cancer cells. Br J Cancer 2003;88(5):796–802.
28. Maeda K, Chung YS, Ogawa Y, et al. Prognostic value of vascular endothelial growth factor expression in gastric carcinoma. Cancer 1996;77(5):858–63.
29. Fondevila C, Metges JP, Fuster J, et al. p53 and VEGF expression are independent predictors of tumour recurrence and survival following curative resection of gastric cancer. Br J Cancer 2004;90(1):206–15.
30. Yao JC, Wang L, Wei D, et al. Association between expression of transcription factor Sp1 and increased vascular endothelial growth factor expression, advanced stage, and poor survival in patients with resected gastric cancer. Clin Cancer Res 2004;10(12 Pt 1):4109–17.
31. Vidal O, Metges JP, Elizalde I, et al. High preoperative serum vascular endothelial growth factor levels predict poor clinical outcome after curative resection of gastric cancer. Br J Surg 2009;96(12):1443–51.
32. Juttner S, Wissmann C, Jons T, et al. Vascular endothelial growth factor-D and its receptor VEGFR-3: two novel independent prognostic markers in gastric adenocarcinoma. J Clin Oncol 2006;24(2):228–40.
33. Shah MA, Ramanathan RK, Ilson DH, et al. Multicenter phase II Study of irinotecan, cisplatin, and bevacizumab in patients with metastatic gastric or gastroesophageal junction adenocarcinoma. J Clin Oncol 2006;24(33):5201–6.
34. Enzinger PC, Ryan DP, Regan EM, et al. Phase II trial of docetaxel, cisplatin, irinotecan, and bevacizumab in metastatic esophagogastric cancer. ASCO Meeting Abstracts. Orlando (FL), August 18, 2008;26(Suppl 15):4552.
35. El-Rayes BF, Zalupski M, Bekai-Saab T, et al. A phase II study of bevacizumab, oxaliplatin, and docetaxel in locally advanced and metastatic gastric and gastroesophageal junction cancers. Ann Oncol 2010;21(10):1999–2004.
36. Shah MA, Jhawer M, Ilson DH, et al. Phase II study of modified docetaxel, cisplatin, and fluorouracil with bevacizumab in patients with metastatic gastroesophageal adenocarcinoma. J Clin Oncol 2011;29(7):868–74.
37. Ohtsu A, Shah MA, Van Cutsem E, et al. Bevacizumab in combination with chemotherapy as first-line therapy in advanced gastric cancer: a randomized, double-blind, placebo-controlled phase III study. J Clin Oncol 2011. [Epub ahead of print].
38. Smyth EC, Enzinger PC, Li J, et al. Bevacizumab (Bev) plus chemotherapy for advanced gastroesophageal adenocarcinoma (GC): Combined U.S. experience. ASCO Meeting Abstracts. Orlando (FL), June 9, 2011;29(Suppl 15):4056.
39. Okines AF, Langley R, Cafferty FH, et al. Preliminary safety data from a randomized trial of perioperative epirubicin, cisplatin plus capecitabine (ECX) with or

without bevacizumab (B) in patients (pts) with gastric or oesophagogastric junction (OGJ) adenocarcinoma. ASCO Meeting Abstracts. Orlando (FL), June 14, 2010;28(suppl 15):4019.

40. Okines AF, Langley RE, Thompson LC, et al. Safety results from a randomized trial of perioperative epirubicin, cisplatin plus capecitabine (ECX) with or without bevacizumab (B) in patients (pts) with gastric or type II/III oesophagogastric junction (OGJ) adenocarcinoma. ASCO Meeting Abstracts. Orlando (FL), June 9, 2011;29(Suppl 15):4092.

41. Prewett M, Huber J, Li Y, et al. Antivascular Endothelial growth factor receptor (fetal liver kinase 1) monoclonal antibody inhibits tumor angiogenesis and growth of several mouse and human tumors. Cancer Res 1999;59(20):5209–18.

42. Spratlin JL, Cohen RB, Eadens M, et al. Phase I pharmacologic and biologic study of ramucirumab (IMC-1121B), a fully human immunoglobulin G1 monoclonal antibody targeting the vascular endothelial growth factor receptor-2. J Clin Oncol 2010;28(5):780–7.

43. Bang YJ, Kang YK, Kang WK, et al. Phase II study of sunitinib as second-line treatment for advanced gastric cancer. Invest New Drugs 2011;29(6):1449–58.

44. Moehler M, Mueller A, Hartmann JT, et al. An open-label, multicentre biomarker-oriented AIO phase II trial of sunitinib for patients with chemo-refractory advanced gastric cancer. Eur J Cancer 2011;47(10):1511–20.

45. Khushalani NI, Fetterly GJ, Iyer RV, et al. Phase I study of sunitinib with irinotecan/5-fluorouracil/leucovorin (FOLFIRI) for advanced gastroesophageal cancers. ASCO Meeting Abstracts. Orlando (FL), June 14, 2010;28(Suppl 15):TPS201.

46. Sebolt-Leopold JS, Herrera R. Targeting the mitogen-activated protein kinase cascade to treat cancer. Nat Rev Cancer 2004;4(12):937–47.

47. Beeram M, Patnaik A, Rowinsky EK. Raf: a strategic target for therapeutic development against cancer. J Clin Oncol 2005;23(27):6771–90.

48. Yang S, Ngo VC, Lew GB, et al. AZD6244 (ARRY-142886) enhances the therapeutic efficacy of sorafenib in mouse models of gastric cancer. Mol Cancer Ther 2009;8(9):2537–45.

49. Kim C, Lee JL, Choi YH, et al. Phase I dose-finding study of sorafenib in combination with capecitabine and cisplatin as a first-line treatment in patients with advanced gastric cancer. Invest New Drugs 2010. [Epub ahead of print].

50. Sun W, Powell M, O'Dwyer PJ, et al. Phase II study of sorafenib in combination with docetaxel and cisplatin in the treatment of metastatic or advanced gastric and gastroesophageal junction adenocarcinoma: ECOG 5203. J Clin Oncol 2010;28(18):2947–51.

51. Mendelsohn J, Baselga J. The EGF receptor family as targets for cancer therapy. Oncogene 2000;19(56):6550–65.

52. Tokunaga A, Onda M, Okuda T, et al. Clinical significance of epidermal growth factor (EGF), EGF receptor, and c-erbB-2 in human gastric cancer. Cancer 1995;75(Suppl 6):1418–25.

53. Dragovich T, McCoy S, Fenoglio-Preiser CM, et al. Phase II Trial of erlotinib in gastroesophageal junction and gastric adenocarcinomas: SWOG 0127. J Clin Oncol 2006;24(30):4922–7.

54. Takehana T, Kunitomo K, Suzuki S, et al. Expression of epidermal growth factor receptor in gastric carcinomas. Clin Gastroenterol Hepatol 2003;1(6):438–45.

55. Lieto E, Ferraraccio F, Orditura M, et al. Expression of vascular endothelial growth factor (VEGF) and epidermal growth factor receptor (EGFR) is an independent prognostic indicator of worse outcome in gastric cancer patients. Ann Surg Oncol 2008;15(1):69–79.

56. Ciardiello F, De Vita F, Orditura M, et al. Cetuximab in the treatment of colorectal cancer. Future Oncol Apr 2005;1(2):173–81.
57. Okines A, Cunningham D, Chau I. Targeting the human EGFR family in esophagogastric cancer. Nat Rev Clin Oncol Aug 2011;8(8):492–503.
58. Chan JA, Blaszkowsky LS, Enzinger PC, et al. A multicenter phase II trial of single-agent cetuximab in advanced esophageal and gastric adenocarcinoma. Annals of Oncology June 1, 2011;22(6):1367–73.
59. Gold PJ, Goldman B, Iqbal S, et al. Cetuximab as second-line therapy in patients with metastatic esophageal adenocarcinoma: a phase II Southwest Oncology Group Study (S0415). J Thorac Oncol Sep 2010;5(9):1472–6.
60. Liu X, Guo WJ, Zhang XW, et al. Cetuximab enhances the activities of irinotecan on gastric cancer cell lines through downregulating the EGFR pathway upregulated by irinotecan. Cancer Chemother Pharmacol Oct 2011;68(4):871–8.
61. Pinto C, Di Fabio F, Siena S, et al. Phase II study of cetuximab in combination with FOLFIRI in patients with untreated advanced gastric or gastroesophageal junction adenocarcinoma (FOLCETUX study). Ann Oncol Mar 2007;18(3):510–7.
62. Pinto C, Di Fabio F, Barone C, et al. Phase II study of cetuximab in combination with cisplatin and docetaxel in patients with untreated advanced gastric or gastro-oesophageal junction adenocarcinoma (DOCETUX study). Br J Cancer 2009;101(8):1261–8.
63. Kim C, Lee JL, Ryu MH, et al. A prospective phase II study of cetuximab in combination with XELOX (capecitabine and oxaliplatin) in patients with metastatic and/or recurrent advanced gastric cancer. Invest New Drugs 2011;29(2): 366–73.
64. Moehler M, Mueller A, Trarbach T, et al. Cetuximab with irinotecan, folinic acid and 5-fluorouracil as first-line treatment in advanced gastroesophageal cancer: a prospective multi-center biomarker-oriented phase II study. Ann Oncol Jun 2011;22(6):1358–66.
65. Rao S, Starling N, Cunningham D, et al. Phase I study of epirubicin, cisplatin and capecitabine plus matuzumab in previously untreated patients with advanced oesophagogastric cancer. Br J Cancer 2008;99(6):868–74.
66. Rao S, Starling N, Cunningham D, et al. Matuzumab plus epirubicin, cisplatin and capecitabine (ECX) compared with epirubicin, cisplatin and capecitabine alone as first-line treatment in patients with advanced oesophago-gastric cancer: a randomised, multicentre open-label phase II study. Ann Oncol 2010;21(11): 2213–9.
67. Okines AF, Ashley SE, Cunningham D, et al. Epirubicin, oxaliplatin, and capecitabine with or without panitumumab for advanced esophagogastric cancer: dose-finding study for the prospective multicenter, randomized, phase II/III REAL-3 trial. J Clin Oncol 2010;28(25):3945–50.
68. Harari D, Yarden Y. Molecular mechanisms underlying ErbB2/HER2 action in breast cancer. Oncogene 2000;19(53):6102–14.
69. Allgayer H, Babic R, Gruetzner KU, et al. c-erbB-2 is of independent prognostic relevance in gastric cancer and is associated with the expression of tumor-associated protease systems. J Clin Oncol 2000;18(11):2201–9.
70. Gravalos C, Jimeno A. HER2 in gastric cancer: a new prognostic factor and a novel therapeutic target. Ann Oncol 2008;19(9):1523–9.
71. Tanner M, Hollmen M, Junttila TT, et al. Amplification of HER-2 in gastric carcinoma: association with topoisomerase IIalpha gene amplification, intestinal type, poor prognosis and sensitivity to trastuzumab. Ann Oncol 2005;16(2): 273–8.

72. Fujimoto-Ouchi K, Sekiguchi F, Yasuno H, et al. Antitumor activity of trastuzumab in combination with chemotherapy in human gastric cancer xenograft models. Cancer Chemother Pharmacol 2007;59(6):795–805.

73. Shah MA, Janjigian YY, Pauligk C, et al. Prognostic significance of human epidermal growth factor-2 (HER2) in advanced gastric cancer: a U.S. and European international collaborative analysis. ASCO Meeting Abstracts. Chicago (IL), June 9, 2011;29(Suppl 15):4014.

74. Krop IE, Beeram M, Modi S, et al. Phase I study of trastuzumab-DM1, an HER2 antibody-drug conjugate, given every 3 weeks to patients with HER2-positive metastatic breast cancer. J Clin Oncol 2010;28(16):2698–704.

75. Barok M, Tanner M, Koninki K, et al. Trastuzumab-DM1 is highly effective in preclinical models of HER2-positive gastric cancer. Cancer Lett 2011;306(2): 171–9.

76. Iqbal S, Goldman B, Fenoglio-Preiser CM, et al. Southwest Oncology Group study S0413: a phase II trial of lapatinib (GW572016) as first-line therapy in patients with advanced or metastatic gastric cancer. Ann Oncol 2011. [Epub ahead of print].

77. LaBonte MJ, Manegold PC, Wilson PM, et al. The dual EGFR/HER-2 tyrosine kinase inhibitor lapatinib sensitizes colon and gastric cancer cells to the irinotecan active metabolite SN-38. Int J Cancer 2009;125(12):2957–69.

78. Wainberg ZA, Anghel A, Desai AJ, et al. Lapatinib, a dual EGFR and HER2 kinase inhibitor, selectively inhibits HER2-amplified human gastric cancer cells and is synergistic with trastuzumab in vitro and in vivo. Clin Cancer Res 2010;16(5): 1509–19.

79. Bjornsti MA, Houghton PJ. The TOR pathway: a target for cancer therapy. Nat Rev Cancer 2004;4(5):335–48.

80. Lang SA, Gaumann A, Koehl GE, et al. Mammalian target of rapamycin is activated in human gastric cancer and serves as a target for therapy in an experimental model. Int J Cancer 2007;120(8):1803–10.

81. Xu DZ, Geng QR, Tian Y, et al. Activated mammalian target of rapamycin is a potential therapeutic target in gastric cancer. BMC Cancer 2010;10: 536.

82. Okamoto I, Doi T, Ohtsu A, et al. Phase I clinical and pharmacokinetic study of RAD001 (everolimus) administered daily to Japanese patients with advanced solid tumors. Jpn J Clin Oncol 2010;40(1):17–23.

83. Doi T, Muro K, Boku N, et al. Multicenter phase II study of everolimus in patients with previously treated metastatic gastric cancer. J Clin Oncol 2010;28(11): 1904–10.

84. Lim T, Lee J, Lee DJ, et al. Phase I trial of capecitabine plus everolimus (RAD001) in patients with previously treated metastatic gastric cancer. Cancer Chemother Pharmacol 2011;68(1):255–62.

85. Birchmeier C, Birchmeier W, Gherardi E, et al. Met, metastasis, motility and more. Nat Rev Mol Cell Biol 2003;4(12):915–25.

86. Comoglio PM, Giordano S, Trusolino L. Drug development of MET inhibitors: targeting oncogene addiction and expedience. Nat Rev Drug Discov 2008;7(6): 504–16.

87. Lee JH, Han SU, Cho H, et al. A novel germ line juxtamembrane Met mutation in human gastric cancer. Oncogene 2000;19(43):4947–53.

88. Smolen GA, Sordella R, Muir B, et al. Amplification of MET may identify a subset of cancers with extreme sensitivity to the selective tyrosine kinase inhibitor PHA-665752. Proc Natl Acad Sci U S A 2006;103(7):2316–21.

89. Janjigian YY, Tang LH, Coit DG, et al. MET expression and amplification in patients with localized gastric cancer. Cancer Epidemiol Biomarkers Prev 2011; 20(5):1021–7.
90. Yap TA, Olmos D, Brunetto AT, et al. Phase I trial of a selective c-MET inhibitor ARQ 197 incorporating proof of mechanism pharmacodynamic studies. J Clin Oncol 2011;29(10):1271–9.
91. Jhawer M, Kindler HL, Wainberg Z, et al. Assessment of two dosing schedules of GSK1363089 (GSK089), a dual MET/VEGFR2 inhibitor, in metastatic gastric cancer (GC): interim results of a multicenter phase II study. ASCO Meeting Abstracts. Orlando (FL), June 8, 2009;27(15S):4502.
92. Eder JP, Shapiro GI, Appleman LJ, et al. A phase I study of foretinib, a multi-targeted inhibitor of c-Met and vascular endothelial growth factor receptor 2. Clin Cancer Res 2010;16(13):3507–16.
93. Saito H, Tsujitani S, Oka S, et al. The expression of transforming growth factor-beta1 is significantly correlated with the expression of vascular endothelial growth factor and poor prognosis of patients with advanced gastric carcinoma. Cancer 1999;86(8):1455–62.
94. Ammanamanchi S, Brattain MG. Restoration of transforming growth factor-beta signaling through receptor RI induction by histone deacetylase activity inhibition in breast cancer cells. J Biol Chem 2004;279(31):32620–5.
95. Fetterly GJ, Brady WE, LeVea CM, et al. A phase I pharmacokinetic (PK) study of vorinostat (V) in combination with irinotecan (I), 5-fluorouracil (5FU), and leucovorin (FOLFIRI) in advanced upper gastrointestinal cancers (AGC). ASCO Meeting Abstracts. Orlando (FL), June 8, 2009;27(15S):e15540.
96. Schwartz GK, Ilson D, Saltz L, et al. Phase II study of the cyclin-dependent kinase inhibitor flavopiridol administered to patients with advanced gastric carcinoma. J Clin Oncol 2001;19(7):1985–92.
97. Schwartz GK, O'Reilly E, Ilson D, et al. Phase I study of the cyclin-dependent kinase inhibitor flavopiridol in combination with paclitaxel in patients with advanced solid tumors. J Clin Oncol 2002;20(8):2157–70.
98. Shah MA, Khanin R, Tang L, et al. Molecular classification of gastric cancer: a new paradigm. Clin Cancer Res 2011;17(9):2693–701.
99. Kang YK, Kang WK, Shin DB, et al. Capecitabine/cisplatin versus 5-fluorouracil/cisplatin as first-line therapy in patients with advanced gastric cancer: a randomised phase III noninferiority trial. Ann Oncol 2009;20(4):666–73.

Endoscopic Mucosal Resection, Endoscopic Submucosal Dissection, and Beyond: Full-Layer Resection for Gastric Cancer with Nonexposure Technique (CLEAN-NET)

Haruhiro Inoue, MD, PhD[a,b,*], Haruo Ikeda, MD[b],
Toshihisa Hosoya, MD[b], Akira Yoshida, MD, PhD[b],
Manabu Onimaru, MD, PhD[b], Michitaka Suzuki, MD[b],
Shin-ei Kudo, MD, PhD[b]

KEYWORDS

- Early gastric cancer • EMR • ESD • CLEAN-NET
- Full-layer resection • Full-thickness resection
- Nonexposure technique

Surgical resection of gastrointestinal cancers is often associated with significant morbidity and mortality. Therefore, methods for endoscopic cancer resection have been sought. With adequate staging techniques, endoscopic resection of early lesions looks promising.[1–5] In surgically resected specimens, intramucosal cancer has an extremely small risk of lymph node metastasis. Therefore, endoscopic resection of mucosal cancer is potentially curable without lymph node dissection. EMR/ESD is a technique of local excision of neoplastic lesions confined to the mucosal layer. However, EMR is a snare-based resection method similar to endoscopic polypectomy. The resected margin is often difficult to control accurately.[6] In contrast, ESD is a knife-based dissection procedure[6–11] in which the resected margin is first

[a] Showa University International Training Center for Endoscopy (SUITE), Digestive Disease Center, Showa University Northern Yokohama Hospital, Yokohama, Japan
[b] Digestive Disease Center, Showa University Northern Yokohama Hospital, Yokohama, Japan
* Corresponding author.
E-mail address: haruinoue777@yahoo.co.jp

Surg Oncol Clin N Am 21 (2012) 129–140
doi:10.1016/j.soc.2011.09.012
1055-3207/12/$ – see front matter © 2012 Elsevier Inc. All rights reserved.

Key Points

- Intramucosal cancer and SM1 cancer (slight sub mucosal invasion) with a low risk of vascular or lymphatic spread with intestinal-type histology are suitable for endoscopic mucosal resection (EMR) and endoscopic submucosal dissection (ESD)

- Chromoendoscopy (indigo carmine spraying) is useful in the stomach to define the lateral margins of tumors during EMR/ESD

- Mucosal lifting by submucosal injection makes EMR/ESD feasible

- Deep ulcer scar in the lesion makes it difficult to resect by EMR/ESD

- Highly scarred lesions can be totally resected by full-layer resection of the gastric wall

- Full-layer resection of gastric wall with non-exposure technique (CLEAN-NET) potentially avoids tumor dissemination

- CLEAN-NET combined with regional lymph node dissection may suggest further application of this procedure to submucosal cancer

---

identified and cut. The major advantage of ESD is that the lateral margin is sufficiently preserved.

This article discusses the efficacy and limitations of EMR/ESD .

BASIC PRINCIPLES OF EMR/ESD

The mucosa and muscularis propria are attached to each other by the loose connective tissue of the submucosa. Submucosal injection creates space between them, which allows resection of the mucosa alone, leaving the muscularis propria layer intact. Saline injection into the submucosal layer is the easiest and most cost-effective technique for separating the layers. Lifting of the mucosal surface can be achieved after correct submucosal injection in any part of the gastrointestinal tract. After a sufficient volume of saline has been injected, the mucosa, including the target lesion, can be safely captured and resected by electrocautery or can be dissected by cutting submucosal tissue with an electrocautery knife (**Fig. 1**).

BRIEF HISTORY OF THE DEVELOPMENT OF EMR/ESD
Choosing the Appropriate Lesions

Intramucosal cancer with no lymph node metastasis is a definite indication for EMR/ESD. Only mucosal lesions with a low risk of vascular or lymphatic spread are appropriate for EMR/ESD. Accumulated data from surgical lymph node dissections revealed that early stage gastric cancer generally has a low risk of lymph node metastasis. Gotoda and colleagues[12] evaluated the risk of nodal metastasis and advocated ESD for selected gastric lesions. Based on these data, properly selected early stage gastric cancers have no risk of lymph node metastasis (95% confidence). Experts in ESD now consider cases of scarring to be the last unsolved issue in ESD.

Endoscopic ultrasonography is often used to assess lesion depth in conjunction with conventional endoscopy. Magnifying endoscopy is useful to evaluate cancer histopathologic types, but is not useful to assess invasion depth. Biopsy before resection should be a routine procedure because poorly differentiated tumors are more likely to invade deeper layers and often metastasize to lymph nodes, and therefore

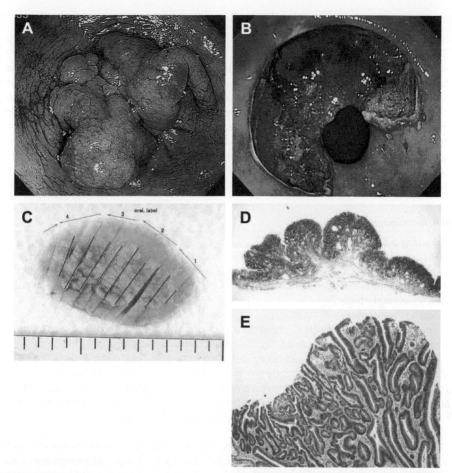

Fig. 1. Early gastric cancer, 0 to I. (*A*) Chromoendoscopic view with indigo carmine dye spray. Large elevated tumor was observed at the antrum. Large nodules in the lesion may suggest submucosal invasion, but upward growth pattern of the tumor cannot exclude the possibility of mucosal cancer. (*B*) Endoscopic view after ESD. Two-thirds circumferential ESD was performed. Distal cut margin of tumor reaches to the duodenum over the pyloric ring. (*C*) Resected specimen. This specimen was cut into multiple 5-mm columns, and was evaluated by microscopy. Red lines show superficial distribution of neoplasia. (*D*) Low-power magnified view. Tumor showed upward growth. Infiltration of the tumor was limited within mucosa. (*E*) Moderately magnified microscopic view. Well-differentiated adenocarcinoma with low-grade atypia.

should be excluded from indications for EMR/ESD. In general, well or moderately differentiated mucosal lesions are considered acceptable targets for EMR/ESD.

Precise evaluation of surgically resected specimens revealed that intestinal-type cancer with slight submucosal invasion (SM1) also has the least risk of lymph node metastasis with no vessel invasion.[12]

Even a flat lesion that contains a poorly differentiated histologic appearance may have a higher risk of invasion beyond the mucosa, and therefore should be resected surgically.[12] Flat lesions with ulcers or scars may have a risk of deeper invasion beyond the mucosa.

Evaluation of Lateral Margins of the Tumor During EMR/ESD

Chromoendoscopy with indigo carmine is useful for defining the lesion before EMR/ESD. The edges of tumor extension may be generally ill defined, particularly with flat lesions. In the stomach, indigo carmine can be used to increase contrast at the interface between normal mucosa and neoplastic lesions. More recently, narrow-band imaging (NBI) magnification endoscopy has been used to distinguish tumor borders from background mucosa by evaluation of surface pattern or vascular pattern.[13–15] Acetic acid is useful to enhance surface patterns. Once fully visualized, it is useful to mark the edges of the lesions before removal and this can be accomplished with cautery from a snare tip a few millimeters outside the border of the lesion. The presence of cautery markings may be helpful in confirming en bloc resection of a lesion and in reorienting the tissue once it has been removed in multiple fragments.

EMR Techniques

EMR using a cap-fitted endoscope

EMR cap (EMR-C) technique[4] is fast, easy to perform, and can be applied to small lesions (<1 cm). Cap refers to an attachment on the distal tip of the forward-viewing endoscope that is made from a transparent plastic material. The EMR-C technique involves several steps.

Step 1: Preparation

In preparation for the EMR-C procedure, a cap is attached to the tip of the forward-viewing endoscope and is fixed tightly with adhesive tape. For the initial session of EMR in the stomach, an obliquely cut, large-capacity cap with a rim (Olympus MAJ297) is most commonly used by fixing it to the tip of the standard-size endoscope to obtain a larger sample. For trimming a residual lesion, a straight-cut, medium-sized cap with a rim (Olympus MH595) is appropriate. All of the items needed for the EMR-C procedure are commercially available in an EMR kit (Olympus).

Step 2: Markings

The mucosal surface that surrounds the margin of the lesion is carefully marked with cautery using the tip of the snare wire or tip of dual knife (Olympus). Markings are positioned 2 mm from the lesion margin. The color enhancement produced by chromoendoscopy disappears within a couple of minutes, and marking by electrocoagulation is therefore essential, especially for a flat lesion.

Step 3: Injection

A diluted epinephrine-saline solution (0.5 mL 0.1% epinephrine solution in 100 mL normal saline) is injected into the submucosa with an injection needle (23-gauge, tip length 4 mm). Puncturing the target mucosa at a sharp angle is important to avoid transmural penetration of the needle tip. The total volume of injected saline depends on the size of the lesion, but it is necessary to inject enough saline to lift up the entire lesion. Usually, more than 20 mL is injected. When saline is accurately injected into the submucosal layer, lifting of the mucosa or its bulging is observed.

Step 4: Prelooping of the snare wire

A specially designed small-diameter snare (with an outer diameter of 1.8 mm; Olympus SD-221L-25) is essential for the prelooping process. The snare wire is fixed along the rim of the EMR-C cap. To create prelooping conditions, moderate suction is first applied to the normal mucosa to seal the outlet of the cap, and the snare wire that passes through the endoscope instrument channel is then opened. The opened snare wire is fixed along the rim of the cap, and the snare's outer sheath sticks up to the rim of the cap.

Step 5: Suction of the target mucosa

With the prelooping position maintained, the lesion is fully captured inside the cap and strangulated by simple closure of the prelooped snare wire. At this stage, the strangulated mucosa looks like a snared polypoid lesion.

Step 6: Resection

The pseudopolyp of the strangulated mucosa is cut using blended current electro-cautery. The resected specimen can be removed by keeping it inside the cap, without using grasping forceps. The smooth surface of the muscularis propria layer is exposed at the bottom of the EMR-induced ulcer.

Step 7: Additional resection

If additional resection is necessary to remove the residual lesion completely, all the stages, including saline injection, should be repeated step by step. The injected saline usually infiltrates and disappears within a few minutes at the initial injection site, so it no longer acts as a cushion between the mucosa and muscle layer. Repeated saline injection is therefore necessary to reduce the risk of perforation.[16]

EMR using a ligating device (EMR-L) is also a popular procedure.[17] In this proce-dure, a ligating device for varices is used to create a pseudopolyp. This procedure is technically easy but the specimen is small and limited. One researcher reported a comparative study of EMR-C and EMR-L. They used a small cap for EMR-C. We routinely use a large cap and, therefore, the resected specimen size is larger than with EMR-L.

ESD

EMR was originally based on snare polypectomy. The size of the specimen resected by EMR is limited to a maximum of around 2 to 3 cm. ESD is a novel technique for endoscopic resection that enables 1-piece resection, even for a superficial and widely spreading tumor. In ESD, first described by Ono and colleagues,[6] a knife activated by electrocautery is used both to cut margins and for submucosal dissection beneath iso-lated mucosa. Devices designed for ESD include the insulation-tip knife, hook knife, dual knife, and flush knife.[6–11] Each knife has specific features for different applica-tions. The authors prefer to use the flush knife because it has an irrigation function through the outer sheath of the knife. The flush knife irrigation system works both as a submucosal injection needle and for irrigation. It is particularly useful for detecting the bleeding point in cases of bleeding.

Triangle-tip knife procedure

The ESD technique using a triangle-tip knife[10] allows removal of the lesion in a single specimen, even for an extended lesion. The triangle-tip knife is a multipurpose device that can be used for marking, cutting, dissecting, and even hemostasis. Using an edge of the triangle-tip knife, the normal mucosa is marked around the lesion. Injection with high-viscosity solution is mandatory for this procedure because it maintains mucosal lifting for a longer duration. The authors use hyaluronic acid for injection. The energy source is an important factor in performing safe ESD. Swift coagulation (ERBE; Vaio) is considered to be the best electrocautery device for the triangle-tip knife. Marginal cutting about 5 mm outside the markings is the next step. The triangle-tip knife hooks the mucosal edge and pulls the target mucosa away from the surface of the muscle layer, and then cuts it by electrocautery. By repeating the process, circumferential incision around the lesion is completed. Submucosal dissection using the tip of a triangle-tip knife is subsequently performed. A hood mounted on the tip of the endo-scope creates a working space beneath the mucosa, and provides countertraction to the tissue in the submucosa. After removal of the mobilized mucosa, complete hemo-stasis is achieved with coagulation forceps.

Which Procedure Should be Used?

Generally, small lesions can be easily excised with the EMR-C procedure. Gastric lesions smaller than 1 cm can be resected by a single session of EMR-C. ESD is used for larger lesions, to perform en bloc mucosal resections. ESD can be used for any lesions regardless of the size and location of the tumor. The only technical limitation of ESD is for gastric lesions with severe scars, which is easily predicted from signs of nonlifting during submucosal saline injection.

Clinical Results and Complications of EMR/ESD in the Stomach

Many reports[18–21] from Japan support clinical validity of ESD for M, N0, or SM1N0 lesions. Other reports from Korea, Europe, and Taiwan also support the clinical feasibility of ESD with acceptable risks.[22–24] Potential complications include bleeding, perforation, and stricture. Bleeding can generally be managed with endoscopic hemostasis using electrocautery forceps. Endoscopic clipping is the last choice to control bleeding from large vessels. Perforation is rare and is treated mainly by endoscopic clipping or conservative management, depending on the size and location of the perforation.[25] Most recently, the Over-The-Scope-clip (Ovesco) is another option for treating perforation. The incidence of delayed perforation is 0.45%, and it should generally be treated by emergency surgery.[26]

In our institution, a total of 679 lesions in 653 cases received EMR or ESD (from April 2001 to December 2011) (**Box 1**). In a series of 653 patients, the author's group used the EMR-C procedure for 181 lesions. No procedure-related death occurred. Perforation occurred in 14 cases (2.0%). In all cases of gastric perforation, the perforated wound was closed using a hemostatic clip. Post-ESD bleeding occurred in 14 cases (2.0%). Bleeding was controlled endoscopically in 13 cases and, in 1 case, it was controlled by angiography. No one required surgery.

FULL-LAYER RESECTION

With the development of various tools for ESD and the improvement in ESD techniques, a gastric lesion in any part and in any size can be safely resected. ESD for a lesion with a severe ulcer scar is one of the major unsolved issues with ESD, because the mucosa of these lesions fails to lift with submucosal injection. In a severely scarred case with signs of nonlifting, it is difficult to identify the correct submucosal plane and

---

Box 1
EMR/ESD for gastric cancer at Showa University Northern Yokohama Hospital, Yokohama, Japan from April 2001 to December 2010

- 653 cases, 679 lesions
- EMR, 181 lesions; ESD, 498 lesions
- No procedure-related death
- Perforation, 14 cases (2.0%). All cases recovered conservatively
- Post-ESD bleeding, 14 cases (2.0%). Bleeding was controlled endoscopically
- Blood transfusion, 5 cases in 14 cases
- Lateral margin(+) or Vertical margin(+) 72 cases
- Local recurrence 11 cases (11/72)

find the perforation. Even when ESD has been successfully performed, resected specimens may have severe heat damage, which results in poor histologic analysis of the lesion. Therefore, a full-thickness resection of the gastric wall for lesions with severe scarring is being studied and developed.

Brief History of Development

Full-layer resection is not a new method. Local resection of gastric lesions during open laparotomy is a basic surgical skill. The size of the resected specimen is smaller than that of a standard gastrectomy, but it still demands a large surgical wound in open surgery. Since the introduction of laparoscopic surgery, a local resection can be done using a linear stapling device through small wounds for trocar sites.

However, direct dissection using a linear stapler often causes severe deformity of the remnant stomach, which potentially causes prolonged gastric emptying. For a small gastric tumor, particularly located along the greater curvature, direct dissection using a linear stapling device is still a quick and technically easy procedure. However, for large tumors and/or tumors located along the lesser curve, a novel technique of full-thickness resection leading to less deformity of the gastric wall is being developed.

Endoscopic and Laparoscopic Full-Thickness Resection

A combined technique of gastrointestinal endoscopy and thoracoscopy/laparoscopy has been reported for the treatment of submucosal tumors (SMT) in the esophagus.[27] This is the first report of combined treatment. In this technique, SMT was pushed out by a balloon on a gastrointestinal endoscope and a pushed-out tumor was enucleated using a thoracoscope. In the stomach, Hiki and colleagues[28] first reported combined laparoscopy and endoscopy surgery for gastrointestinal stromal cell tumors (GIST). In their technique, with the combined use of both optics, adjacent gastric wall close to a GIST was circumferentially cut in a full-layer fashion. After resection of the GIST, the fully opened gastric wall was closed with laparoscopic manual suturing or a laparoscopic lineal stapler. The major advantage of this technique is to reduce the resected area of gastric wall, which may avoid stomach deformity caused by wide-area, full-layer resection. Kitano and Shiraishi[29] reported an improved technique. In this technique, overlying serosa is cut first, allowing easy mobilization of SMT and less deformity of the stomach. These 2 methods are open techniques that expose the gastric lumen, but their application is limited to SMT, which may not increase the risk of peritoneal dissemination.

Full-thickness resection for gastric cancer under laparoscopic and endoscopic guidance was first performed by Abe and colleagues.[30] It was combined with lymph node dissection. It may open a new era in the treatment of gastric cancer, but there are major criticisms of this technique. Gastric lumen is completely opened to the peritoneal cavity (**Fig. 2**). To some degree, gastric contents flow and contaminate the clean peritoneal cavity. This contamination may be acceptable for resection of nonepithelial tumors (GIST), but is not acceptable for the treatment of epithelial tumors. The potential risk of peritoneal dissemination can not be ignored in this technique.

It is necessary to develop and establish full-layer resection with a nonexposure method. We developed and reported a combination of laparoscopic and endoscopic approaches for neoplasia using a nonexposure technique.[31]

CLEAN-NET

CLEAN-NET is a combined laparoscopic and endoscopic approach for neoplasia with a nonexposure technique. When endoscopic resection is combined with laparoscopic

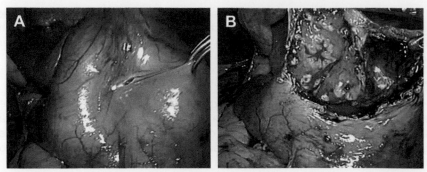

Fig. 2. Conventional exposed technique for full-thickness resection in the stomach. (*A*) Using insulation-tipped (IT) knife 2 (Olympus) inserted through peroral endoscopy full-layer gastric wall dissection was performed. The insulation tip of the IT knife 2 was observed as a white ball at the cutting edge. (*B*) Laparoscopic view. Gastric wall including cancer was resected. The gastric lumen was eventually exposed to the peritoneal cavity. A major criticism of this technique is that gastric contents often flow into peritoneal cavity during the procedure, which may cause viable cancer cell seeding to peritoneal cavity.

surgery, full-layer resection is easy to perform. However, a major criticism of the procedure is that gastric content may flow into the peritoneal cavity through the open gastric wall incision. It is impossible to completely prevent the risk of cancer cell dissemination, so a nonexposure technique needs to be developed. CLEAN-NET was developed by using a seromuscular incision, preserving the continuity of the mucosa, which works as a barrier (a clean net).

By using a seromuscular incision, mucosa that surrounds the full-layer specimen is stretched and maintains a sufficient epithelial margin around the cancer tissue. The size of the resected muscle layer is approximately the same as the epithelial lesion, so gastric deformity can be kept to a minimum.

Technical Details of CLEAN-NET

Marking around the lesion
Lateral spread of mucosal cancer is carefully identified with indigo carmine chromoendoscopy and NBI magnification endoscopic. By spraying of indigo carmine, a cancerous lesion is often enhanced as an uncolored area. NBI magnifying endoscopic observation allows any irregularity of the surface structure and neovascularity to be observed. In mucosal cancer, the surface pattern becomes irregular and abnormal vessels are often observed.[13–15] After identification of a superficial extension, endoscopic markings are made on the mucosa surrounding the lesion with an electrocautery knife (**Fig. 3**A). The markings are made approximately 5 mm from the cancer margin. This process is similar to ESD.

Fixation of mucosa and muscle layer
The mucosal and seromuscular layers are loosely attached to each other with submucosal connective tissue. A positional gap often exists to some degree between the 2 layers. The mucosal layer must therefore be fixed to the seromuscle layer with full-layer stitches using 4 stay sutures, which is performed with laparoscopic guidance. The position of the stay sutures is also controlled by endoscopic vision from inside the stomach, at or outside the markings (see **Fig. 3**B).

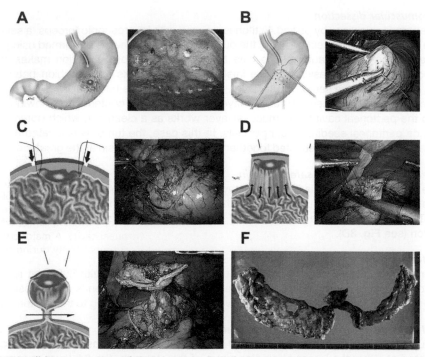

Fig. 3. Full-layer resection of the gastric wall with the nonexposure technique, combining laparoscopic and endoscopic approaches for neoplasia with the nonexposure technique (CLEAN-NET). In this procedure, both serosa and muscle layer were selectively dissected using a laparoscopic electrocautery knife. Preserved mucosal layer works as a mechanical barrier (CLEAN-NET) between the gastric lumen and peritoneal cavity, which potentially avoids peritoneal cavity contamination by gastric content. (*A*) Marking around the lesion. Superficial extension of mucosal cancer is generally identified by both chromoendoscopy with indigo carmine and careful observation using NBI magnification. After identification of superficial extension, endoscopic markings are placed on the surrounding mucosa of the lesion with the electrocautery knife. This process is equal to ESD. (*B*) Fixation of mucosa and muscle layer. The mucosal layer and seromuscular layer are loosely attached to each other with submucosal connective tissue. A positional gap often occurs between the 2 layers. The mucosal layer is fixed onto the seromuscular layer using 4 stay sutures, which are introduced using laparoscopic vision and controlled by endoscopic vision from inside the stomach. (*C*) Seromuscular dissection. By pulling 4 stitches upward with laparoscopic forceps, selective seromuscular dissection outside the 4 stitches is performed using a laparoscopic electrocautery knife. The continuity of the mucosal layer remains intact, preventing the gastric contents from flowing out into the peritoneal cavity. The mucosal layer works as a clean net, which potentially avoids peritoneal seeding of cancer cells. In this case, the tumor was located at the greater curve, and was resected together with the lymphatic basin. (*D*) Increasing the cancer-free safety margin. A full-layer specimen is lifted by 4 stay sutures. Mucosa surrounding the full-layer specimen is also pulled up toward the specimen. This process allows a wider cancer-free margin around a full-thickness lesion. (*E*) Full-layer resection using a mechanical stapler. The lesion can be resected together with intragastric contents without exposing the mucosal surface to the peritoneal cavity. (*F*) Resected specimen. Full-layer specimen is resected together with its lymphatic basin. If the tumor is located at either the lesser curve or greater curve of the stomach, a full-layer specimen including local tumor can be resected together with dissected lymphatic basin.

Seromuscular dissection

In laparoscopic view, by pulling 4 stitches upward with laparoscopic forceps, a selective seromuscular dissection along the outside of the 4 stitches is performed using an laparoscopic electrocautery knife (see **Fig. 3**C). Submucosal injection makes this process technically easier because injected solution works as a cushion between the mucosa and the seromuscular layer. In this method, the mucosal layer maintains its continuity. The preserved mucosal layer prevents gastric contents from flowing out into the peritoneal cavity. The mucosal layer works as a clean net, which potentially avoids peritoneal seeding of cancer cells. In this case, the tumor was located at the greater curve, and was resected together with its lymphatic basin at the greater curve.

Obtaining a cancer-free safety margin

The full-layer specimen is lifted by 4 stay sutures. Mucosa surrounding the full-layer specimen is also pulled up, together with the full-layer specimen.

This process allows a wide mucosal cancer-free margin around a full-thickness lesion (see **Fig. 3**D).

Full-layer cut

Using a mechanical stapler, a cancerous full-layer specimen with sufficient lateral mucosal margin is cut and taken out (see **Fig. 3**E). Gastric lumen is not exposed to the peritoneal cavity, which potentially avoids cancer cells seeding to the peritoneum.

Full-layer specimen and related lymph node

A full-layer specimen is resected en bloc with its lymphatic basin. If the tumor is located at either the lesser or greater curve of the stomach, the full-layer specimen involving the local tumor can be resected together with the lymphatic basin at the tumor site. If the tumor is located at the anterior or posterior wall of the stomach, lymphatic flow to the sentinel node is often complicated. In contrast, lymph node dissection on both sides (lesser curve and major curve), like conventional surgery, may cause ischemia of the stomach, so selection of the lymph node dissection side is mandatory at this stage. The resected specimen is stretched onto a rubber board. All lymph nodes are also picked up from the resected specimen and are carefully evaluated by pathologists.

Clinical results of CLEAN-NET

CLEAN-NET was applied to 24 consecutive cases. Sixteen cases had gastric cancer and 8 cases had GIST. In 22 cases, the procedure was completed successfully with

---

Box 2
Clinical results of CLEAN-NET

Male/female ratio = 14:2

Age: 66.2 years (45–82 years)

Blood loss: 18 mL (trace to 92 mL)

Oral intake starts 4.5 days after procedure

Pathology:

  Mucosal cancer: 8 cases

  SM1: 3 cases

  Massive submucosal invasion (SM2): 5 cases

good clinical results. In 1 case, surgical repair was necessary because of incomplete closure of the resected line by the linear stapling device. In another case, additional surgery was necessary to improve gastric deformity. Clinical data from 16 cases of gastric cancer are summarized in **Box 2**. No clinical sign of recurrence was identified in any of the cases.

SUMMARY

EMR/ESD has been widely accepted as a curative treatment of early gastric cancer. Now there are 2 major treatment options (EMR/ESD and laparoscopic surgery) for early gastric cancer. But as a treatment of T1M, N0 cancer with deep ulcer scar, EMR/ESD is technically difficult to complete and laparoscopic surgery may be a treatment option. For such a case, the authors have developed a combined endoscopic and laparoscopic procedure to complete full-thickness resection of the gastric wall. CLEAN-NET allows full-layer gastric wall resection to be completed with less deformity and little leakage of gastric content into the abdominal cavity. CLEAN-NET is potentially combined with lymph node dissection of the lymphatic basin, and may become another treatment option for T1N0 gastric cancer.

REFERENCES

1. Deyhle P, Sauberli H, Noesch HJ, et al. Endoscopic "jumbo biopsy" in the stomach with a diathermy loop. Acta Hepatogastroenterol (Stuttg) 1974; 21:228–32.
2. Tada M, Murakami A, Karita M, et al. Endoscopic resection of early gastric cancer. Endoscopy 1993;25:445–50.
3. Inoue H, Endo M. Endoscopic esophageal mucosal resection using a transparent tube. Surg Endosc 1990;4:198–201.
4. Inoue H, Takeshita K, Hori H, et al. Endoscopic mucosal resection with a capfitted panendoscope for esophagus, stomach, and colon mucosal lesions. Gastrointest Endosc 1993;39:58–62.
5. Lambert R. Diagnosis of esophagogastric tumors. Endoscopy 2004;36:110–9.
6. Ono H, Kondo H, Gotoda T, et al. Endoscopic mucosal resection for treatment of early gastric cancer. Gut 2001;48:225–9.
7. Yamamoto H, Yube T, Isoda N, et al. A novel method of endoscopic mucosal resection using sodium hyaluronate. Gastrointest Endosc 1999;50:251–6.
8. Oyama T, Kikuchi Y. Aggressive endoscopic mucosal resection in the upper GI tract – Hook knife EMR method. Minim Invasive Ther Allied Technol 2002;11: 291–5.
9. Yahagi N, Fujishiro M, Iguchi M, et al. Theoretical and technical requirements to expand EMR indications. Dig Endosc 2003;15:S19–21.
10. Inoue H, Satoh Y, Sugaya S, et al. Endoscopic mucosal resection for early-stage gastrointestinal cancers. Best Pract Res Clin Gastroenterol 2005;19:871–87.
11. Toyonaga T, Man-i M, Fujita T, et al. Retrospective study of technical aspects and complications of endoscopic submucosal dissection for laterally spreading tumors of the colorectum. Endoscopy 2010;42:714–22.
12. Gotoda T, Yanagisawa A, Sasako M, et al. Incidence of lymph node metastasis from early gastric cancer: estimation with a large number of cases at two large centers. Gastric Cancer 2000;3:219–25.
13. Nakayoshi T, Tajiri H, Matsuda K, et al. Narrow-band imaging system with magnifying endoscopy for early gastric cancer: correlation of vascular pattern with histopathology. Endoscopy 2004;36:1080–4.

14. Yao K, Anagnostopoulos GK, Ragunath K. Magnifying endoscopy for diagnosing and delineating early gastric cancer. Endoscopy 2009;41:462–7.
15. Yokoyama A, Inoue H, Minami H, et al. Novel narrow-band imaging magnifying endoscopic classification for early gastric cancer. Dig Liver Dis 2010;42:704–8.
16. Inoue H, Kawano T, Tani M, et al. Endoscopic mucosal resection using a cap: technique for use and preventing perforation. Can J Gastroenterol 1999;13: 477–80.
17. Nwakakwa V, Fleischer D. Endoscopic mucosal resection of the esophagus: band ligation technique. Gastrointest Endosc Clin N Am 2001;11:479–88.
18. Sanomura Y, Oka S, Tanaka S, et al. Clinical validity of endoscopic submucosal dissection for submucosal invasive gastric cancer: a single-center study. Gastric Cancer 2011. [Epub ahead of print].
19. Goto O, Fujishiro M, Kodashima S, et al. Outcomes of endoscopic submucosal dissection for early gastric cancer with special reference to validation of curability criteria. Endoscopy 2009;41:118–22.
20. Isomoto H, Shikuwa S, Yamaguchi N, et al. Endoscopic submucosal dissection for early gastric cancer: a large-scale feasibility study. Gut 2009;58:331–6.
21. Gotoda T. Endoscopic resection of early gastric cancer: the Japanese perspective. Curr Opin Gastroenterol 2006;22:561–9.
22. Chung IK, Lee JH, Lee SH, et al. Therapeutic outcomes in 1000 cases of endoscopic submucosal dissection for gastric neoplasms: Korean ESD Study Group multicenter study. Gastrointest Endosc 2009;69:1228–35.
23. Probst A, Pommer B, Golger D, et al. Endoscopic submucosal dissection in gastric neoplasia-experience from a European center. Endoscopy 2010;42: 1037–44.
24. Lee IL, Wu CS, Tung SY, et al. Endoscopic submucosal dissection for early gastric cancers: experience from endoscopic center in Taiwan. J Clin Gastroenterol 2008;42:42–7.
25. Fujishiro M, Yahagi N, Kakushima N, et al. Successful nonsurgical management of perforation complicating endoscopic submucosal dissection of gastric intestinal epithelial neoplasms. Endoscopy 2006;38:1001–6.
26. Hanaoka N, Uedo N, Ishihara R, et al. Clinical features and outcomes of delayed perforation after endoscopic submucosal dissection for early gastric cancer. Endoscopy 2010;42:1112–5.
27. Izumi Y, Inoue H, Endo M. Combined endoluminal-intracavitary thoracoscopic enucleation of leiomyoma of the esophagus. A new method. Surg Endosc 1996;10:457–8.
28. Hiki N, Yamamoto Y, Fukunaga T, et al. Laparoscopic and endoscopic cooperative surgery for gastrointestinal stromal tumor dissection. Surg Endosc 2008;22: 1729–35.
29. Kitano S, Shiraishi N. Minimally invasive surgery for gastric tumors. Surg Clin N Am 2005;85:151–64.
30. Abe N, Mori T, Takeuchi H, et al. Successful treatment of early gastric cancer by laparoscopy-assisted endoscopic full-thickness resection with lymphadenectomy. Gastrointest Endosc 2008;68:1220–4.
31. Inoue H, Minami H, Ogata N, et al. How can we decide treatment of early stage gastric cancer? Choosing EMR/ESD, laparoscopic surgery or another. Endoscopia Digestiva 2009;21:749–54.

Laparoscopic Resection for Gastric Carcinoma: Western Experience

Vivian E. Strong, MD

KEYWORDS

- Gastric cancer • Laparoscopic gastrectomy
- Gastric carcinoma • Western experience
- Minimally invasive gastrectomy

LAPAROSCOPIC APPROACHES FOR GASTRIC CARCINOMA: WESTERN EXPERIENCE

Gastric cancer represents an important worldwide health concern and is the second leading cause of cancer deaths worldwide.[1] Although the incidence is higher in Eastern countries (78 cases per 100,000 in Japan compared with 10 cases per 100,000 in the United States),[2] it still remains the fourth leading cause of cancer deaths in the United States, and each year, more than 21,000 Americans are diagnosed with gastric cancer and almost 11,000 die of the disease.[3]

There has been much speculation regarding differences in outcome for patients who have gastric cancer in the Eastern versus Western world, especially considering the greater frequency of early gastric cancer in Eastern countries and their higher incidence of distal, intestinal-type tumors. This situation is in contrast to the Western experience of tumors that are more often identified at an advanced stage and are more often proximal in location or at the gastroesophageal junction and more often of diffuse-type histology. Among other factors, these differences have contributed to a unique cohort of patients and experience in the Western staging/evaluation of gastric cancer and in the application of minimally invasive approaches for treatment. This review summarizes the current state of laparoscopic approaches for the staging and treatment of gastric adenocarcinoma for patients presenting in Western countries, with their associated unique presentation, comorbidities, and outcomes.

The author has nothing to disclose.
Gastric and Mixed Tumor Service, Department of Surgery, Memorial Sloan-Kettering Cancer Center, Weill Medical College of Cornell University, 1275 York Avenue, H-1217, New York, NY 10065, USA
E-mail address: strongv@mskcc.org

Surg Oncol Clin N Am 21 (2012) 141–158
doi:10.1016/j.soc.2011.09.010
1055-3207/12/$ – see front matter © 2012 Elsevier Inc. All rights reserved.

Rational for Diagnostic Laparoscopy and Cytology

The current National Comprehensive Cancer Network Practice Guidelines in Oncology emphasize the importance of managing gastric carcinoma via a multidisciplinary approach,[4] including a team of dedicated oncologists specializing in gastroenterology, surgical oncology, medical oncology, pathology, and radiology for upper gastrointestinal cancers. Diagnosis requires upper endoscopy and biopsy for tissue diagnosis. Computed tomography (CT) scanning and endoscopic ultrasonography (EUS) are important tests for staging. For patients who are found to have locally advanced disease, defined as T3 or greater or node-positive via EUS and CT evaluation, treatment recommendations include multimodality therapy.[5] Before neoadjuvant treatment can begin, completion staging of these patients requires diagnostic laparoscopy to detect radiologically occult visible M1 disease, found in up to 40% of patients.[6,7,8,9]

Diagnostic laparoscopy not only identifies visible, subradiographic M1 disease but also allows for collection of cytologic peritoneal washings for evaluation. Positive peritoneal cytology (positive for cancer cells) is now included in the American Joint Committee on Cancer staging system as consistent with metastatic (M1) disease.[10] This strategy is based on studies showing that despite complete (R0) resection of a gastric carcinoma, patients with positive peritoneal cytology have a median survival of months that parallels visible metastatic disease. There are almost no patients who have survived longer than 3 years with positive peritoneal cytology.[11,12,13,14,15]

Based on previous studies from our institution and others, positive peritoneal cytology is an independent predictor of outcome in patients with gastric cancer despite R0 resection.[11,12,14,15,16]

From Memorial Sloan-Kettering Cancer Center, a review of more than 650 patients with gastric carcinoma who had no radiographic evidence of metastatic disease on CT imaging underwent diagnostic laparoscopy, and 31% were found to have occult (subradiographic) peritoneal disease.[17] The highest risk for peritoneal disease was found in patients with visible nodal involvement on CT scan or those with tumors involving the entire stomach (linitis plastica) or tumors at the gastroesophageal junction. Since then, other studies evaluating the predictive value of EUS have shown additional effectiveness in selecting patients at higher risk of having occult metastatic disease for diagnostic laparoscopy. Power and colleagues[18] analyzed 94 patients with localized gastric cancer who underwent EUS and staging laparoscopy and found that those with EUS results of early gastric cancer, defined as T1 or T2 and N0, had a significantly lower risk of peritoneal disease than those with locally advanced disease, defined as ultrasonic T3 or T4 or N positive tumors (4% vs 25%). Based on these data, we routinely recommend laparoscopy to rule out occult metastases only for those with locally advanced disease.

Therefore, at our cancer center, diagnostic laparoscopy is used as part of our standard staging evaluation to identify occult peritoneal metastases for patients with locally advanced gastric carcinoma. These patients undergo separate staging laparoscopy with cytologic washings before initiation of neoadjuvant chemotherapy. Patients with positive peritoneal cytology are treated with palliative chemotherapy.

Evolving Experience with Minimally Invasive Gastric Cancer Surgery

The only potentially curative treatment of gastric carcinoma is surgical resection. An appropriate cancer operation requires at least a D1 dissection, although most academic centers throughout the West advocate a D2 dissection.[19,20] Although a laparotomy is the most common approach for surgical resection of gastric carcinoma, many controversies exist regarding the ideal surgical strategy, including whether and when a laparoscopic approach is appropriate. Laparoscopic approaches for gastric cancer have been accepted slowly, largely because of the advanced technical skills required, combined with the necessary oncologic principles that must be met for oncologically appropriate resection, including the gastric resection and adequate lymphadenectomy. Because this disease is rarely seen except at high-volume cancer centers in the United States, the experience in the United States is therefore still limited.

Overall, the Eastern experience has been instrumental in leading the way to the standardization and acceptance of minimally invasive approaches, in large part because of a higher volume of gastric cancer and early-stage disease that has facilitated the application of this approach. Despite these advances, the laparoscopic approach is still relatively new. In 1992, Ohgami and colleagues[21] reported the first laparoscopic wedge resection for the treatment of early gastric cancer. In 1994, Kitano and colleagues[22] performed the first laparoscopy-assisted distal gastrectomy (LADG) with a modified D1 lymph node dissection for the treatment of early gastric cancer.

Since then, many reports have shown both the feasibility and oncologic adequacy of minimally invasive approaches when performed by surgeons with high-volume exposure and advanced laparoscopic skills, mostly in Eastern countries. However, laparoscopic gastrectomy for all stages of gastric cancer is gradually emerging in the West, although this progress has been slowed by differences in the natural history of gastric adenocarcinoma in the East compared with the West. It was not until 1999 that Azagra and colleagues[23] reported the first laparoscopic total gastrectomy for stomach cancer followed by the first totally LADG with Billroth II anastomosis for cancer in 1993. **Table 1** summarizes the published experience with laparoscopic surgery for the treatment of gastric cancer.

Table 1
Major Western series for minimally invasive approaches for resection of gastric carcinoma

Study	Total Patients (N)	Laparoscopic Surgery (n)	Open Surgery (n)	Operative Mortality in the Laparoscopic Group (n/N [%])	Lymph Nodes Removed (n)[a]
Huscher 2005[24]	59	30	29	1/30 (3.3)	30 ± 14.9
Carboni 2005[61]	20	20	0	0/20 (0)	23–47 (range)
Dulucq 2005[62,63]	52	24	28	0/24 (0)	24 ± 12
Weber 2003[64]	25	12	13	0/12 (0)	8 (4–14)
Feliu 2007[65]	23	23	0	0/23 (0)	21.3 ± 5
Pugliese 2007[66]	147	48	99	1/48 (2.1)	30 ± 7 (D1) 32 ± 7 (D2)
Varela 2006[71]	36	15	21	0/15 (0)	15 ± 9
Anderson 2007[67]	7	7	0	0/7 (0)	24 (17–30) (median and range)
Orsenigo 2009[68]	34	34	0	0/34 (0)	31 ± 10
Reyes 2001[27]	36	18	18	0/18 (0)	8 (4–14)
Azagra 2006[69]	101	91	0	5/91 (5.5)	17 ± 5 (D1) 37 ± 14 (D2)
Besozzi 2007[70]	24	24	0	3/24 (12.5)	25 (15–50)
Strong 2009[28]	60	30	30	0	18
Guzman 2009[29]	80	32	48	0	26

[a] Mean ± standard deviation, unless otherwise noted.

Huscher and colleagues[24] have the only Western prospective randomized trial to date looking at laparoscopic gastrectomy for all resectable stages of gastric cancer. In their study, 59 patients with a gastric cancer were prospectively randomized to open subtotal or laparoscopic-assisted subtotal gastrectomy. Patients were matched for pTNM stage. Five-year overall survival rates of 59% versus 56%, respectively, and 5-year disease-free survival rates of 57% versus 55% showed oncologic equivalency of the 2 approaches along with the additional benefits of the laparoscopic approach such as decreased length of hospital stay, reduced blood loss, and earlier resumption of oral intake (**Table 2**).

In the United States, the first group to publish their experience with laparoscopic gastrectomy for gastric cancer was Reyes and colleagues in 2001.[27] In this retrospective case-matched study, there were no significant differences in extent of lymph node dissection or in intraoperative complications between groups. The laparoscopic approach required a significantly longer operative time (4.2 vs 3.0 hours for the open group), likely because of the learning curve of this procedure. However, in the laparoscopic versus open groups, there was less blood loss, an earlier return to bowel function, decreased postoperative ileus, and a significantly reduced hospital stay (6.3 vs 8.6 days).

The largest published series of minimally invasive gastrectomy in North America to date comes from Memorial Sloan-Kettering Cancer Center and City of Hope. In the Memorial Sloan-Kettering Cancer Center experience, a total of 60 patients were evaluated, including 30 minimally invasive gastrectomies and 30 open gastrectomies (**Table 3**). Median operative time for the laparoscopic approach was 270 minutes (range 150–485 minutes) compared with 126 minutes (range 85–205 minutes) in the open group ($P<.01$). Hospital length of stay after laparoscopic gastrectomy was 5 days (range 2–26 days), compared with 7 days (range 5–30 days) in the open group ($P = .01$). Postoperative intravenous narcotic use was shorter for laparoscopic patients, with a median of 3 days (range 0–11 days) compared with 4 days (range 1–13 days) in the open group ($P<.01$). Postoperative late complications were significantly higher for the open group ($P = .03$). Short-term recurrence-free survival and margin status was similar with adequate lymph node retrieval in both groups (**Fig. 1**). This series concluded that laparoscopic gastrectomy for carcinoma is comparable with the open approach with regard to oncologic principles of resection, with equivalent margins and adequate lymph node retrieval, showing technical feasibility and similar short-term recurrence-free survival (see **Table 3**).[28]

In the City of Hope experience, a total of 78 consecutive patients were evaluated, including 30 minimally invasive gastrectomies and 48 open gastrectomies (**Tables 4 and 5**).[29] All laparoscopic resections had negative resection margins and 15 or more lymph nodes retrieved in the surgical specimen, with no difference in the number of lymph nodes retrieved by laparoscopic or open approaches (24 ± 8 vs 26 ± 15, $P = .66$). The minimally invasive procedures were associated with decreased blood loss (200 vs 383 mL, $P = .0009$) and length of stay (7 vs 10 days, $P = .0009$), but increased operative time (399 vs 298 minutes, $P<.0001$). Overall complication rate for the minimally invasive group was lower although not statistically significant.

In a recent meta-analysis of Eastern and Western randomized, controlled trials (RCTs) and high-quality observational studies comparing the laparoscopic and open subtotal gastrectomies, 38 studies published between 2000 and 2009 that met thoughtfully considered validated eligibility criteria and included 6 RCTs and 32 high-quality nonrandomized controlled trials allowed for comparison of a total of 3055 patients with 1658 undergoing laparoscopic subtotal gastrectomy (54%) and 1397 (46%) undergoing open subtotal gastrectomy. Results from that study are summarized in **Table 6** and show no significant difference in the postoperative

Table 2
Prospective, randomized studies in the East and West comparing laparoscopic-assisted and open gastrectomy for gastric carcinoma

Study	Procedures	Patients (LADG/ODG), n	Mean Operative Time (LADG/ODG), min ± SD	Mean Blood Loss (LADG/ODG), mL ± SD	Oral Intake Resumed (LADG/ODG), Mean Postoperative Days ± SD	Complications (LADG/ODG), %
Kitano et al,[25] 2002	LADG vs ODG	14/14	227 ± 7/171 ± 13	117 ± 30/258 ± 53	5.3 ± 1.5/4.5 ± 0.3	14.3/28.6
Hayashi et al,[26] 2005	LADG vs ODG	14/14	378 ± 97/235 ± 71	327 ± 245/489 ± 301	3.5 ± 0.8/5.4 ± 1.2	35.7/57.1
Lee 2005[Lee 2005b]	LADG vs ODG	24/23	319 ± 16.2/190.4 ± 39.1	336.4 ± 180.3/294.4 ± 156.3	5.3 ± 1.4/5.7 ± 2.8	12.5/43.5
Huscher et al,[24] 2005	LADG vs ODG	30/29	196 ± 21/168 ± 29	229 ± 144/391 ± 136	5.1 ± 0.5/7.4 ± 2.0	23.3/27.6
Kim et al,[41] 2008	LADG vs ODG	82/82	253 ± 49/171 ± 27	112 ± 85/267 ± 155	3.8 ± 0.7/4.1 ± 0.5	22-Sep

Abbreviations: LADG, laparoscopy-assisted distal gastrectomy; ODG, open distal gastrectomy; SD, standard deviation.

Table 3
Operative characteristic and complications for laproscopic versus open gastrectomy patients from MS/CCC series

Median (Range)	Laparoscopic (n = 30)	Open (n = 30)	P Value
Procedure			
Billroth II	20	22	NS
Roux-en-Y	10	8	—
Operation time (min)	270 (150–485)	126 (85–205)	<0.01
Estimated blood loss (cc)	200 (50–800)	150 (100–850)	NS
Length of stay (d)	5 (2–26)	7 (5–30)	0.01
Intravenous narcotic use (d)	3.0 (0–11)	4.0 (1–13)	<0.01
Early complications (<30 d)	8 (26%)	13 (43%)	0.07
Late complications	0 (0%)	6 (20%)	0.03

Abbreviation: NS, not significant.
Data From Strong VE, Devaud N, Allen PJ, et al. Laoroscopic gastronomy versus open gastractomy for adenocarcinomus: a case-control study. Ann Surg Oncol 2007;16(6):1507–13.

mortality, or major surgical complications. The retrieval of lymph nodes was significantly higher in the open gastrectomy group by 3.9 nodes (95% confidence interval [CI] 2.4–5.4, $P<.001$), although the odds of having fewer than 15 lymph nodes harvested were comparable, suggesting similar staging and oncologic equivalency.[30]

Laparoscopy has been shown to be a safe option for the treatment of gastric cancer, which compares favorably with open gastrectomy in short-term outcomes. Laparoscopic approaches may result in a clinically insignificant but lower lymph node retrieval, especially for more advanced gastric cancers that are undergoing more extended lymphadenectomy, although these early results may be related to learning curve issues. The long-term oncologic impact of this approach is unclear and although numerous studies have clearly established this approach as a valid and effective treatment of early gastric cancer in the East, the approach must be further validated in the West for more advanced proximal tumors in patients with

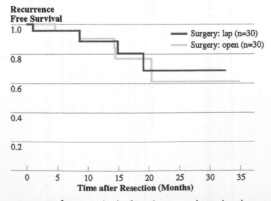

Fig. 1. Short-term recurrence-free survival of patients undergoing laparoscopic versus open resection of gastric carcinoma. (*Data from* Strong VE, Devaud N, Allen PJ, et al. Laparoscopic gastrectomy versus open gastrectomy for adenocarcinoma: a case-control study. Ann Surg Oncol 2009;16(6):1507–13.)

Table 4
Short term outcomes of laproscopic and open gastrectomies

	Laparoscopic (n = 30)	Open (n = 48)	P Value
Surgery time (min), mean (SD)	399 (85)	298 (77)	<.0001
Estimated blood loss, median (range)	200 (50–900)	383 (50–2600)	.0009
Length of stay (d), median (range)	7 (3–32)	10 (3–67)	.0009
Weight loss at 1 mo (%), mean	6.77	7.74	.4195
30-d mortality (n)	0	1	.4262
Conversions (n)	1	—	—
Complications (n)	9	22	.161
Arrhythmia (n)	2	8	—
Anastomotic leak (n)	1	0	—
Duodenal stump leak (n)	1	0	—

Abbreviation: SD, standard deviation.
Data From Guzman EA, Pisazz A, Lee B, et al. Totally Laproscopic Gastric rescetion with extended Lymphadenectomy for Gastric Adenocarcinoma. Ann Surg Oncol 2009;16:2218–23.

higher body mass indexes (calculated as weight in kilograms divided by the square of height in meters) and associated comorbidities.

Indications and Contraindications

When applying any new technology to a cancer operation, caution with regard to appropriate indications must be applied. Contraindications are relative and evolving, determined by multifactorial criteria, including the technical expertise of the surgeon and experience with advanced minimally invasive techniques as well as the relative achievement of the learning curve, which is largely predicated by the understanding and volume of experience with the disease. A solid understanding of gastric cancer, its modes of presentation, differences in the natural history of diffuse and intestinal types, and overall differences in biologic behavior of this heterogeneous disease is paramount to the appropriate selection of the optimal technical approach to provide an oncologic sound, safe, and appropriate operation for your patient. Relative contraindications for a surgeon who is early in their learning curve include patients with a high body mass index, those with more advanced gastric tumors, and those requiring associated en bloc resections of surrounding invaded structures. As with any new technology, it is critical to keep sight of the most important goals for the patient with a low threshold for

Table 5
Oncologic outcomes from city of hope series of gastrectomies

	Laparoscopic (n = 30)	Open (n = 48)	P Value
Negative margin (n [%])	30 (100)	47 (98)	.4262
Closest margin (cm), mean (SD)	3.8 (1.82)	3.6 (2.35)	.7695
Number of lymph nodes (mean [SD])	24.4 (8.22)	25.7 (14.54)	.6579

Abbreviation: SD, standard deviation.
Data From Adenocarcinoma Guzman EA, Pisazz A, Lee B, et al. Totally Laproscopic Gastric rescetion with extended Lymphadenectomy for Gastric Adenocarcinoma. Ann Surg Oncol 2009;16:2218–23.

Table 6
Meta-analysis of RCT and high-quality observational studies comparing laparoscopic and open distal gastrectomy: odds ratios less than 1 or a positive weighted mean difference (WMD) favors the laparoscopic group

Outcome	Odds Ratio/WMD	95% CI	P Value
Mortality	0.64	0.23–1.8	0.39
Overall complications	0.59	0.47–0.74	<0.001
Major surgical complications	0.84	0.56–1.27	0.42
Minor surgical complications	0.62	0.46–0.83	0.001
Medical complications	0.49	0.31–0.77	0.002
Harvested lymph nodes	3.9	2.4–(-) 5.4	<0.001
Operative time (min)	48.3	34.2–62.4	<0.001
Blood loss (mL)	119	91–(-) 147	<0.001
Hospital stay (d)	3.6	2.6–(-) 4.5	<0.001

Data from Viñuela EF, Gonen M, Brennan MF, et al. Laparoscopic versus open distal gastrectomy for gastric cancer: a meta-analysis of randomized controlled trials and high quality non-randomized studies. Ann Surg, in press; and Parkin DM, Bray F, Ferlay J, et al. Global cancer statistics, 2002. CA Cancer J Clin 2005;55(2):74–108.

conversion to an open approach. A technically and oncologically equivalent operation must be provided for the patient via the minimally invasive approach.

The safety of the patient is always considered above the technical approach. For this reason, patients with multiple or severe comorbidities such as severe cardiac or pulmonary disease, who may benefit from a shorter anesthetic time, may not be well served by minimally invasive approaches. In addition, patients undergoing gastrectomy after neoadjuvant treatment tend to have more technically complicated operations that should be cautiously approached early in one's learning curve. Also, patients who have undergone multiple previous laparotomies and have extensive adhesions are not good candidates for the laparoscopic approach. Clearly, thin and healthy patients with early gastric cancers in the distal half of the stomach are the most feasible and approachable tumors for a laparoscopic approach. As the learning curve progresses and the surgeon's understanding of the biologic behavior of the disease matures, indications may be broadened. After an extensive learning curve with distal, early gastric cancers in the East, the indications are now expanding to advanced gastric cancers, and a randomized, prospective trial is under way in South Korea to definitively answer this question.

Results and Outcomes

Since the first published report of laparoscopic gastrectomy for gastric cancer in 1994, by Kitano and colleagues, there have been an increasing number of reports of results and outcomes for the laparoscopic approach compared with the open approach, mostly from literature in the East, particularly from Japan and Korea. Because much controversy remains about comparisons of gastric cancer in the East and the West, Eastern-derived data should be extrapolated cautiously to Western patients.[31]

Perioperative factors

In a recent meta-analysis of RCT and high-quality observational studies by Viñuela and colleagues,[30] various factors comparing the laparoscopic and open approaches were compared. Operative time was found to take on average 48 minutes longer via the laparoscopic approach compared with the open procedure. Some studies suggest that this difference is related to learning curve issues. Operative blood loss was also found to be lower after laparoscopic gastrectomy, although the clinical relevance of minimal differences in blood loss is debated. In the previously mentioned meta-analysis, the reduction was on average 120 mL.

Other factors, including less postoperative pain, postoperative ileus, earlier oral intake and ambulation, and better postoperative respiratory function, have been reported in retrospective clinical series, case-control studies, and RCTs comparing laparoscopic and open gastrectomy.[25,26,28,32,33,34,35,36,37,38]

The outcome of length of stay has been lower in many Western series reported; however, Eastern studies do not report similar reductions in hospital stay. Practice differences in Eastern compared with Western hospitals may partly account for these differences. In the recent meta-analysis mentioned earlier the investigators analyzed this outcome and found that hospital stay was significantly reduced by more than 3 days after LADG compared with the conventional open procedure **Table 7**.[30]

Quality of life

An important goal of performing less invasive operations is to improve a patient's quality of life. This is a particularly difficult outcome to measure, because many factors are involved, including a patient's understanding of their disease, the possible need for neo-adjuvant therapy, the need for total versus subtotal gastrectomy, and the occurrence of postoperative complications or recurrence, which may be unrelated to the technique used. Long-term quality-of-life studies of open gastrectomy show a postoperative decline of functional outcome that stabilizes, and slowly improves, between 6 and 12 months after surgery.[39] However, in many cases, symptoms may still be troublesome. In 1 study, of 162 patients who underwent open radical gastrectomy, 1 year after their operation, 32.7% had regular or poor appetite, 28,8% had decreased the amount of food they ingested, and 25% had a weight loss greater than 10 kg.[40] There is good evidence showing that quality of life can be improved with the laparoscopic approach. An RCT from South Korea compared laparoscopic-assisted and open distal gastrectomy for early gastric cancer. A total of 164 patients were randomized and quality of life was evaluated up to 3 months after surgery using validated questionnaires. Significantly better scores were found in the laparoscopic-assisted arm, including physical, emotional, and social factors and global quality-of-life score was better. Specific areas were also improved, such as pain, appetite, sleep, diet, and body image.[41]

Postoperative morbidity and mortality

Postoperative complication rates after LADG (<30 days) range between 10% and 20% in Eastern country studies.[42,43] Western country studies report slightly higher morbidity rates, in the 20% to 30% range,[24,28] which may be related to an older cohort of patient with increased comorbidities in Western patients. Whether these figures compare favorably with the open technique is still controversial. The meta-analysis cited previously, which included all published RCTs to date and a selection of high-quality observational studies and included more than 3000 patients, found a highly significant 40% reduction in overall complications, as well as significant reductions in the minor surgical complication and medical complication categories. This finding differs from Eastern reports; in the recent RCT from the Korean Laparoscopic Gastrointestinal Surgery Study Group a nonsignificant ($P = .14$) 28% reduction in the complication rate was observed.[42]

Perioperative complications

Complications that occur during and after gastrectomy are not necessarily specific to the technique used. However, for the laparoscopic approach, unexpected

Table 7
Postoperative recovery outcomes in a selection of observational studies and RCTs comparing laparoscopic (Lap) and open (Op) gastrectomy (bold type indicates statistical significance)

			Lap	Op	Lap	Op	Lap	Op
Observational studies								
Adachi [2]	2000	49 / 53	3.9	4.5	5	5.7	NR	NR
Shimizu [3]	2000	21 / 31	2.5	3.3	7.2	6.3	1.3	1.7
Yano [4]	2001	24 / 35	2.7	3.6	4.5	5.6	1.3	2.3
Dulucq [5]	2005	16 / 17	2.9	5.8	NR	NR	2.5	5.8
Naka [6]	2005	20 / 22	2.1	3.1	4.7	5.1	2.7	4
Lee SI [7]	2006	136 / 120	3.8	4.4	3.9	5.7	NR	NR
Nunobe [8]	2007	39 / 51	2.3	2.7	NR	NR	NR	NR
Lee WJ [9]	2008	34 / 34	2.9	4.9	NR	NR	NR	NR
Song [10]	2008	44 / 31	3.3	4.4	5.8	6.4	NR	NR
Lee JH [11]	2009	106 / 105	3.4	3.9	4.6	5.4	NR	NR
Randomized controlled trials								
Kitano [12]	2002	14 / 14	2.9	3.9	5.3	4.5	1.8	2.6
Hayashi [13]	2005	14 / 14	3.1	3.9	3.5	5.4	NR	NR
Lee [14]	2005	24 / 23	3.7	3.8	5.3	5.7	NR	NR
Huscher [15]	2005	30 / 29	NR	NR	5.1	7.4	NR	NR
Kim [16]	2008	82 / 82	3.4	3.6	3.8	4.1	NR	NR

Abbreviation: NR, not reported.

intraoperative events constitute the major reason for conversion to open gastrectomy. Most are associated with the use of dissection devices or the direct handling of organs by assistants with retractors,[44] some of them away from the operative field. Therefore an experienced surgical team has to be aware of these potential issues. Factors associated with a higher risk of intraoperative events include patients with higher body mass index and more extensive lymphadenectomies.

The incidence of these complications is low. One retrospective study from Korea calculated a 2.6% rate of intraoperative complications. Fifty-six percent were bleeding events, all requiring conversion to open surgery.[45] In the meta-analysis mentioned earlier, 63% of the conversions to open surgery were related to intraoperative bleeding events.[30] Common sources of bleeding are the right gastroepiploic vessels during the dissection of the infrapyloric area and from the common hepatic and splenic arteries during lymphadenectomy.[44,45] Injuries to the pancreas while performing lymph node dissection or lacerations of the distal esophagus during laparoscopic total gastrectomy, if suspected, should prompt conversion to allow for better assessment.

Anastomotic leakage Anastomotic leak must be carefully considered after every gastric resection, whether open or laparoscopic. Disruption of the anastomosis is clinically apparent in approximately 1% to 2% of laparoscopic subtotal gastrectomies and in 5% to 15% of laparoscopic total gastrectomies with a Roux-en-Y esophagojejunal anastomosis.[24,42] The higher leak rate observed after total gastrectomy is related to the connection of the more friable esophagus to jejunum. Typically an anastomotic leak or fistula presents as onset of fever, tachycardia, abdominal pain, and distension between the fourth and seventh postoperative day, but a more insidious clinical picture is possible, so the concern for this event must be considered and evaluated based on clinical signs and symptoms in combination with relevant laboratory values and radiographic studies. If possible, radiologic tests should be performed to confirm the clinical diagnosis if present. An upper gastrointestinal series with water-soluble contrast is helpful in locating the disruption and determining if it is well contained or if it opens freely to the peritoneal cavity. A careful endoscopy is an alternative for a negative esophagogram or a patient not able to swallow. CT imaging is also a useful radiologic test.

Bleeding Postoperative hemorrhage can be seen in approximately 1% of patients.[42] Gastrointestinal bleeding from staple or suture lines can often be managed nonoperatively; however, intra-abdominal bleeding can be potentially life-threatening. The surgeon should have a low threshold for reexploration for suspected bleeding if clinically indicated. After laparoscopic gastrectomy, one must in addition consider postoperative bleeding from the laparoscopic port sites, particularly the specimen extraction site. For open and laparoscopic approaches, postoperative pseudoaneurysms, although extremely rare, can be the source of significant bleeding and may be evident only from CT scan and confirmed by angiography. The treatment of choice is selective embolization at the time of angiography if possible.

Wound complications Wound complications in the laparoscopic setting are uncommon and occur in approximately 2% of patients. The wound most frequently affected is the one used for extraction of the specimen because of its larger size, greater manipulability, and higher potential for contamination. The correct administration of preoperative antibiotics is recommended because they have proved to decrease the rate of wound infection after clean-contaminated surgical interventions, although this has not been specifically established for laparoscopic gastrectomy. Other useful preventive measures are the extraction of the specimen in a retrieval bag, the use of wound protective sheaths, and the extraction of potentially contaminated material through inserted ports. The infection is usually superficial and can be treated on an outpatient basis with removal of a few skin sutures and dressing changes. Oral antibiotics may be required if there are signs of cellulitis in the surrounding skin.

Incisional hernias are less frequent for patients undergoing laparoscopic resections; however, an adequate technique of fascial closure is the single most important preventive measure to avoid port-site hernias. Closure of the larger ports sites (>12 mm) using a fascia closure device is preferable.

Long-term complications

Anastomotic strictures are infrequent after laparoscopic gastrectomy but have been reported as high as 18% after laparoscopic total gastrectomy.[46,47,48,49] They present with early satiety and vomiting in the case of distal gastrectomy or progressive dysphagia after total gastrectomy. Diagnosis is made via an upper gastrointestinal series and endoscopy. In general, strictures are mild and can be treated endoscopically with balloon dilations. Strictures that develop after an anastomotic leak can be more severe and difficult to treat, requiring multiple endoscopic procedures, which may include balloon dilations, stricture section, steroid injection, and the use of expandable stents.

Small bowel obstruction secondary to adhesion formation is not a trivial problem after open gastrectomy, with a reported incidence that varies between 3% and 11%.[50,51,52] About half of these patients require a reoperation for this reason. A reduced incidence of adhesive ileus after laparoscopic procedures is an increasing observation, because longer follow-ups are being reported for diverse laparoscopic operations. This finding has been attributed to the less inflammatory and immunologic peritoneal reaction induced by the laparoscopic surgery[53,54] and to the lower degree of peritoneal trauma inherent to less invasive procedures. A recent systematic study regarding small bowel obstruction and abdominal surgery that included more than 400,000 procedures in total found that the laparoscopic approach was associated with a significantly lower incidence of bowel obstruction for cholecystectomy, gynecologic procedures, and colorectal surgery[55]; gastrectomies were not included. On the other hand, no difference in the incidence of small bowel obstruction between open and laparoscopic colorectal interventions was found in a recent Cochrane meta-analysis.[39] A reduced incidence of obstructive adhesions associated with laparoscopic gastrectomy has been reported in a few small comparative studies, but evidence is still inconclusive.

Postoperative mortality after laparoscopic gastrectomy is less than 1% and is comparable with the mortality of the open procedure, as reported by our recent meta-analysis.[30] The similar mortality found for laparoscopic and open operations is expected because major features of the surgical procedure such as the extent of gastric resection, lymphadenectomy, and reconstruction are all technically similar and encompass the major source of possible postoperative morbidity. This observation was confirmed in the meta-analysis cited earlier, in which the odds of developing serious complications are similar for the laparoscopic and open group.[30]

Learning Curve

The learning curve for laparoscopic gastrectomy for gastric cancer is steep, and outcomes to consider include operative time, complications, and equivalent oncologic resection. Many factors affect the learning process, including intrinsic technical challenges associated with a particular operation such as total gastrectomy and creation of the esophagojejunal anastomosis compared with the relatively more facile gastrojejunostomy associated with a distal gastrectomy. Others factors relate to surgeon training, experience, and dexterity. Hospital environment may also influence the learning curve, including the characteristics and volume of patients treated, surgical equipment, and surgical team.

Because this process is multifactorial and difficult to address, there are few reports addressing this topic. Because Eastern countries have the greatest experience based on high incidence of gastric cancer, the most informative 2 studies on the topic come from Japan and Korea. In 1 study, a gastric surgeon with an experience of more than 1000 open gastrectomies, but with no previous laparoscopic exposure, was trained for 2 months in laparoscopic techniques and then performed 102 laparoscopic distal gastrectomies with Billroth II reconstruction. His experience was divided in 2 groups (50 early cases, 52 late cases) and compared with 71 patients who underwent open distal gastrectomy in the same period. For the latter 52 cases, operative time was shorter (190 vs 230 minutes, $P<.001$), more lymph nodes were retrieved (30 vs 25 mean nodes, $P = .02$), and fewer complications were observed (4 vs 13 events, $P = .03$) than in the early laparoscopic group. However, results did not match those of the open group (mean operative time = 154 minutes; mean harvested nodes = 38 nodes).[56] Another similar study compared 100 patients who underwent LADG with 67 patients operated by the conventional approach. The laparoscopic group was divided in 5 20-patient groups. After 60 cases no conversions were observed and the operative time was similar to the conventional group (227 vs 232 minutes).[57] These and other studies[58,59,60] suggest a learning curve of 50 to 60 cases for LADG, although it has to be underlined that these results are limited by the type of patients and procedures included and they may not reflect the learning curve of patients with more advanced disease requiring standard D2 dissection, which constitutes most patients seen in Western countries. One study found that after learning LADG for early gastric cancer a new threshold in the learning curve was involved if more advanced cases were included or more extensive lymphadenectomies were performed (**Box 1**).[59]

Box 1
Factors affecting the learning curve of laparoscopic gastrectomy
Procedure Factors
Number and complexity of intracorporeal steps
Total versus subtotal gastrectomy
Extent of lymphadenectomy
Early versus locally advanced tumor
Method of anastomosis
Technique standardization
Robotic assistance
Surgeon Factors
Previous experience with laparoscopic surgery
Previous experience with the open technique
Manual dexterity
Environment/Hospital Factors
Patient characteristics
Obesity and comorbidities and previous abdominal operations
Number of patients (ie, frequency of the operation)
Surgical equipment
Surgical team
Experience of other members of the surgical team

Summary and Future Applications

Open gastrectomy with negative margins and a minimal dissection of 15 lymph nodes for staging purposes constitutes an appropriate approach for surgical treatment of gastric adenocarcinoma regardless of technique used. A solid understanding of the disease process and heterogeneity of gastric cancer and variations in the natural history related to histology type, location, and genetic factors in the context of a multi-disciplinary team dedicated to the individualized treatment of a patient with gastric cancer is essential. Once a defined and accurate staging and plan have been determined, the minimally invasive approach to resecting gastric cancer can be assessed. As experience and expertise of oncologic surgeons in the minimally invasive approach to gastric resection for cancer increases, laparoscopic approaches clearly provide benefits for well-selected patients who are appropriate for the application of this technique. For surgeons with oncologic and advanced minimally invasive experience, a laparoscopic gastrectomy with lymphadenectomy provides at least equivalent resection outcomes to the open approach with no proven compromise in disease-free survival or long-term survival based on preliminary studies.

Although the learning curve is steep, the advantages of the minimally invasive approach, including quicker recovery for the patient, less blood loss, and at least equivalent or fewer perioperative complications, should encourage surgical oncologists to expand the indications for this approach. Although the threshold for conversion to an open approach should be low, particularly in cases where there are concerns about a patient's suitability for this approach based on previous operations or health, concerns over local resectability, the definition of anatomy, or the surgeon's comfort level, it seems that the laparoscopic approach is an acceptable procedure for appropriately selected patients with equivalent oncologic outcomes. Until more mature long-term follow-up data on the treatment of advanced gastric cancer with minimally invasive approaches are defined in the West, in which local clearance has been an issue in the open gastrectomy setting, it is recommended that minimally invasive approaches be limited to those patients with well-staged T1 and T2N0 adenocarcinomas, as defined by CT scanning and EUS, particularly in centers that do not treat a large volume of gastric cancers, until experience with the technique expands. In addition, it is recommended that such procedures in the West be performed by surgeons with advanced laparoscopic skills, as well as an understanding of and training in the oncologic approach to gastric cancer. As indications for laparoscopic-assisted gastrectomy continue to expand for more advanced tumors and with data from additional prospective studies, oncologically appropriate application of laparoscopic gastrectomy for all stages of gastric adenocarcinoma will be more clearly defined.

ACKNOWLEDGMENTS

I would like to thank Dr Eduardo Vinuela for his kind assistance in creating several of the tables presented and for his assistance in drafting 2 sections of this article.

REFERENCES

1. Parkin DM, Bray F, Ferlay J, et al. Global cancer statistics, 2002. CA Cancer J Clin 2005;55(2):74–108.
2. Ahmad SA, Choi EA, Rodgers SE, et al. Hepatobiliary cancers. In: Feig BW, Bergner DH, Fhrman GH, editors. The MD Anderson surgical oncology handbook. 4th edition. Philadelphia: Lippincott William & Wilkins; 2006. p. 320–66.

3. Jemal A, Siegel R, Ward E, et al. Cancer statistics, 2008. CA Cancer J Clin 2008; 58(2):71–96.
4. National Comprehensive Cancer Network (NCCN) clinical practice guidelines in oncology: Gastric Cancer (V.2.2010). 2010, National Comprehensive Cancer Network, NCCN. org.
5. Cunningham D, Allum WH, Stenning SP, et al. Perioperative chemotherapy versus surgery alone for resectable gastroesophageal cancer. N Engl J Med 2006; 355(1):11–20.
6. Asencio F, Aguiló J, Salvador JL, et al. Video-laparoscopic staging of gastric cancer. A prospective multicenter comparison with noninvasive techniques. Surg Endosc 1997;11(12):1153–8, 3–6.
7. Burke EC, Karpeh MS, Conlon KC, et al. Laparoscopy in the management of gastric adenocarcinoma. Ann Surg 1997;225(3):262–7.
8. D'Ugo DM, Persiani R, Caracciolo F, et al. Selection of locally advanced gastric carcinoma by preoperative staging laparoscopy. Surg Endosc 1997;11(12): 1159–62.
9. Possik RA, Franco EL, Pires DR, et al. Sensitivity, specificity, and predictive value of laparoscopy for the staging of gastric cancer and for the detection of liver metastases. Cancer 1986;58(1):1–6.
10. American Joint Committee on Cancer. 7th edition. New York (NY): Springer; 2010.
11. Bando E, Yonemura Y, Takeshita Y, et al. Intraoperative lavage for cytological examination in 1,297 patients with gastric carcinoma. Am J Surg 1999;178(3):256–62.
12. Bentrem D, Wilton A, Mazumdar M, et al. The value of peritoneal cytology as a preoperative predictor in patients with gastric carcinoma undergoing a curative resection. Ann Surg Oncol 2005;12(5):347–53.
13. Bonenkamp JJ, Songun I, Hermans J, et al. Prognostic value of positive cytology findings from abdominal washings in patients with gastric cancer. Br J Surg 1996;83(5):672–4.
14. Burke EC, Karpeh MS Jr, Conlon KC, et al. Peritoneal lavage cytology in gastric cancer: an independent predictor of outcome. Ann Surg Oncol 1998;5(5):411–5.
15. Kodera Y, Yamamura Y, Shimizu Y, et al. Peritoneal washing cytology: prognostic value of positive findings in patients with gastric carcinoma undergoing a potentially curative resection. J Surg Oncol 1999;72(2):60–4 [discussion: 64–5].
16. Fukagawa T, Katai H, Saka M, et al. Significance of lavage cytology in advanced gastric cancer patients. World J Surg 2010;34(3):563–8.
17. Sarela AI, Lefkowitz R, Brennan MF, et al. Selection of patients with gastric adenocarcinoma for laparoscopic staging. Am J Surg 2006;191:134–8.
18. Power DG, Schattner MA, Gerdes H, et al. Endoscopic ultrasound can improve the selection for laparoscopy in patients with localized gastric cancer. J Am Coll Surg 2009;208:173–8.
19. Kelsen DP. Postoperative adjuvant chemoradiation therapy for patients with resected gastric cancer: intergroup 116. J Clin Oncol 2000;18(Suppl 21):32S–4S.
20. Macdonald JS, Smalley SR, Benedetti J, et al. Chemoradiotherapy after surgery compared with surgery alone for adenocarcinoma of the stomach or gastroesophageal junction. N Engl J Med 2001;345:725–30.
21. Ohgami M, Otani Y, Kumai K, et al. Curative laparoscopic surgery for early gastric cancer: five years experience. World J Surg 1999;23(2):187–92.
22. Kitano S, Iso Y, Moriyama M, et al. Laparoscopy-assisted Billroth I gastrectomy. Surg Laparosc Endosc 1994;4(2):146–8.
23. Azagra JS, Goergen M, De Simone P, et al. Minimally invasive surgery for gastric cancer. Surg Endosc 1999;13:351–7.

24. Huscher CG, Mingoli A, Sgarzini G, et al. Laparoscopic versus open subtotal gastrectomy for distal gastric cancer: five-year results of a randomized prospective trial. Ann Surg 2005;241(2):232–7.
25. Kitano S, Shiraishi N, Fujii K, et al. A randomized controlled trial comparing open vs laparoscopy-assisted distal gastrectomy for the treatment of early gastric cancer: an interim report. Surgery 2002;131(Suppl 1):S306–11.
26. Hayashi H, Ochiai T, Shimada H, et al. Prospective randomized study of open versus laparoscopy-assisted distal gastrectomy with extraperigastric lymph node dissection for early gastric cancer. Surg Endosc 2005;19(9):1172–6.
27. Reyes CD, Weber KJ, Gagner M, et al. Laparoscopic vs open gastrectomy: a retrospective review. Surg Endosc 2001;15:928–31.
28. Strong VE, Devaud N, Allen PJ, et al. Laparoscopic versus open subtotal gastrectomy for adenocarcinoma: a case-control study. Ann Surg Oncol 2009;16(6):1507–13.
29. Guzman EA, Pigazzi A, Lee B, et al. Totally laparoscopic gastric resection with extended lymphadenectomy for gastric adenocarcinoma. Ann Surg Oncol 2009;16(8):2218–23.
30. Viñuela EF, Gonen M, Brennan MF, et al. Laparoscopic versus open distal gastrectomy for gastric cancer: a meta-analysis of randomized controlled trials and high quality non-randomized studies. Ann Surg. [Epup print ahead].
31. Strong VE, Song KY, Park CH, et al. Comparison of gastric cancer survival following R0 resection in the United States and Korea using an internationally validated nomogram. Ann Surg 2010;251(4):640–6.
32. Adachi Y, Shiraishi N, Shiromizu A, et al. Laparoscopy-assisted Billroth I gastrectomy compared with conventional open gastrectomy. Arch Surg 2000;135(7):806–10.
33. Yano H, Monden T, Kinuta M, et al. The usefulness of laparoscopy-assisted distal gastrectomy in comparison with that of open distal gastrectomy for early gastric cancer. Gastric Cancer 2001;4(2):93–7.
34. Mochiki E, Kamiyama Y, Aihara R, et al. Laparoscopic assisted distal gastrectomy for early gastric cancer: five years' experience. Surgery 2005;137(3):317–22.
35. Kim MC, Kim KH, Kim HH, et al. Comparison of laparoscopy-assisted by conventional open distal gastrectomy and extraperigastric lymph node dissection in early gastric cancer. J Surg Oncol 2005;91(1):90–4.
36. Ziqiang W, Feng Q, Zhimin C, et al. Comparison of laparoscopically assisted and open radical distal gastrectomy with extended lymphadenectomy for gastric cancer management. Surg Endosc 2006;20(11):1738–43.
37. Tanimura S, Higashino M, Fukunaga Y, et al. Respiratory function after laparoscopic distal gastrectomy–an index of minimally invasive surgery. World J Surg 2006;30(7):1211–5.
38. Song KY, Kim SN, Park CH. Laparoscopy-assisted distal gastrectomy with D2 lymph node dissection for gastric cancer: technical and oncologic aspects. Surg Endosc 2008;22(3):655–9.
39. Wu CW, Chiou JM, Ko FS, et al. Quality of life after curative gastrectomy for gastric cancer in a randomised controlled trial. Br J Cancer 2008;98(1):54–9.
40. Wu CW, Hsieh MC, Lo SS, et al. Quality of life of patients with gastric adenocarcinoma after curative gastrectomy. World J Surg 1997;21(7):777–82.
41. Kim YW, Baik YH, Yun YH, et al. Improved quality of life outcomes after laparoscopy-assisted distal gastrectomy for early gastric cancer: results of a prospective randomized clinical trial. Ann Surg 2008;248(5):721–7.
42. Kim HH, Hyung WJ, Cho GS, et al. Morbidity and mortality of laparoscopic gastrectomy versus open gastrectomy for gastric cancer: an interim report–

a phase III multicenter, prospective, randomized trial (KLASS Trial). Ann Surg 2010;251(3):417–20.

43. Kim MC, Kim W, Kim HH, et al. Risk factors associated with complication following laparoscopy-assisted gastrectomy for gastric cancer: a large-scale Korean multicenter study. Ann Surg Oncol 2008;15(10):2692–700.

44. Kim MC, Choi HJ, Jung GJ, et al. Techniques and complications of laparoscopy-assisted distal gastrectomy (LADG) for gastric cancer. Eur J Surg Oncol 2007; 33(6):700–5.

45. Ryu KW, Kim YW, Lee JH, et al. Surgical complications and the risk factors of laparoscopy-assisted distal gastrectomy in early gastric cancer. Ann Surg Oncol 2008;15(6):1625–31.

46. Jeong GA, Cho GS, Kim HH, et al. Laparoscopy-assisted total gastrectomy for gastric cancer: a multicenter retrospective analysis. Surgery 2009;146(3): 469–74.

47. Lee SE, Ryu KW, Nam BH, et al. Technical feasibility and safety of laparoscopy-assisted total gastrectomy in gastric cancer: a comparative study with laparoscopy-assisted distal gastrectomy. J Surg Oncol 2009;100(5):392–5.

48. Kachikwu EL, Trisal V, Kim J, et al. Minimally invasive total gastrectomy for gastric cancer: a pilot series. J Gastrointest Surg 2011;15(1):81–6.

49. Jeong O, Park YK. Intracorporeal circular stapling esophagojejunostomy using the transorally inserted anvil (OrVil) after laparoscopic total gastrectomy. Surg Endosc 2009;23(11):2624–30.

50. Sugimachi K, Korenaga D, Tomikawa M, et al. Factors influencing the development of small intestinal obstruction following gastrectomy for early gastric cancer. Hepatogastroenterology 2008;55(82–83):496–9.

51. Inaba T, Okinaga K, Fukushima R, et al. Prospective randomized study of two laparotomy incisions for gastrectomy: midline incision versus transverse incision. Gastric Cancer 2004;7(3):167–71.

52. Kodera Y, Sasako M, Yamamoto S, et al. Identification of risk factors for the development of complications following extended and superextended lymphadenectomies for gastric cancer. Br J Surg 2005;92(9):1103–9.

53. Jung IK, Kim MC, Kim KH, et al. Cellular and peritoneal immune response after radical laparoscopy-assisted and open gastrectomy for gastric cancer. J Surg Oncol 2008;98(1):54–9.

54. Saba AA, Kaidi AA, Godziachvili V, et al. Effects of interleukin-6 and its neutralizing antibodies on peritoneal adhesion formation and wound healing. Am Surg 1996;62(7):569–72.

55. Barmparas G, Branco BC, Schnuriger B, et al. The incidence and risk factors of post-laparotomy adhesive small bowel obstruction. J Gastrointest Surg 2010; 14(10):1619–28.

56. Yoo CH, Kim HO, Hwang SI, et al. Short-term outcomes of laparoscopic-assisted distal gastrectomy for gastric cancer during a surgeon's learning curve period. Surg Endosc 2009;23(10):2250–7.

57. Kunisaki C, Makino H, Yamamoto N, et al. Learning curve for laparoscopy-assisted distal gastrectomy with regional lymph node dissection for early gastric cancer. Surg Laparosc Endosc Percutan Tech 2008;18(3):236–41.

58. Zhang X, Tanigawa N. Learning curve of laparoscopic surgery for gastric cancer, a laparoscopic distal gastrectomy-based analysis. Surg Endosc 2009;23(6): 1259–64.

59. Jin SH, Kim DY, Kim H, et al. Multidimensional learning curve in laparoscopy-assisted gastrectomy for early gastric cancer. Surg Endosc 2007;21(1):28–33.

60. Kim MC, Jung GJ, Kim HH. Learning curve of laparoscopy-assisted distal gastrectomy with systemic lymphadenectomy for early gastric cancer. World J Gastroenterol 2005;11(47):7508–11.
61. Carboni F, Lepaine P, Santoro, et al. Laproscopic surgery for gastric cancer: preliminary experience. Gastric cancer 2005;8:75–7.
62. Dulucq JL, Wintringer P, Stabilini C, et al. Laproscopic and open geatric resections for malignant lesions: a prospective comprative study. Surg Endosc 2005; 19:933–8.
63. Dulucq JL, Wintringer P, Perrisat J, et al. Completely laproscopic total and partial gastrectomty for bening and malignant diseases: a single institute's prospective analysis. JAm coll surg 2005;200:191–7.
64. Weber KJ, Reyes CD, Gagner M, et al. Comprasion of laproscopic and open gastrectomy for malignant diseases. Surg Endosc 2003;17:968–71.
65. Feliu X, Besora P, Claveria R, et al. Laproscopic treatment of gastric tumors. J Laparoendosc Adv Surg Tech A 2007;17:147–52.
66. Pugliese R, Maggioni D, Sansonna F, et al. Total and subtotal laproscopic gastrectomy for adenocarcinoma. Surg Endosc 2007;21:21–7.
67. Anderson C, Ellenhorn J, Hellan m, et al. Pilot series of robot-assisted laproscopic subtotal gastrectomy with extended lymphadenectomy for gastric cancer. Surg Endosc 2007;21:1662–6.
68. Orsenigo E, Staudacher C. Sentinel node mapping during laproscopic distal gastrectomy for gastric cancer. Surg Endosc 2009;23:919.
69. Azagra Js, Ibanez-Aguirre JF, Gorgen M, et al. Long-term results of laproscopic extended surgery in advanced gastric cancer: a series of 101 patients. Hepatogastroenterology 2006;5353:304–8.
70. Besozzi A, Bessozzi S, Lanza V, et al. Laproscopic treatment gastric cancer with advanced techniques: technial notes and follow-up. Chir ital 2007;59:63–7.
71. Varela JE, Hiyashi M, Nguyen T, et al. Comparison of laparoscopic and open gastrectomy for gastric cancer. Am J Surg 2006;192(6):837–42.

POSTSCRIPT

The following article is an addition to Lung Cancer, the October 2011 issue of *Surgical Oncology Clinics of North America* (Volume 20, Issue 4).

Molecular Markers for Incidence, Prognosis, and Response to Therapy

Betty C. Tong, MD, MHS, David H. Harpole Jr, MD*

KEYWORDS

• Lung cancer • Prognostication • Molecular markers

With more than 1.2 million cases diagnosed annually, lung cancer is the leading cause of cancer mortality worldwide.[1,2] The majority of lung cancer diagnoses are made at advanced stages (III-IV), where the mainstay of treatment is chemotherapy and/or radiation. For early-stage (I-II) lung cancer, surgery is the mainstay of treatment, sometimes in conjunction with adjuvant chemotherapy.

Clinicians optimally should prescribe a course of therapy that is tailored to individual patients and their comorbid conditions to provide best possible outcomes. If patients are considered medically operable, appropriate therapy should include surgical resection for patients with stage I, II, and selected IIIA disease. For the minority of patients with early-stage disease who are not suitable for or refuse surgery, tumor ablative strategies may be used as an alternative to surgery. Adjuvant therapy should be considered in patients with nodal metastasis (N1 and N2) and now for patients with stages Ib and IIa as well. This includes both traditional chemotherapeutic agents as well as molecular targeted agents. With recent advances in genetic, molecular, and proteomic profiling of lung tumors, clinicians can offer treatment that is tailored to individuals and their tumors, with the objective of maximizing long-term survival.

Currently, tumor stage is the most reliable prognostic indicator of long-term survival for patients diagnosed with lung cancer. Recently, the International Association for the Study of Lung Cancer analyzed 67,725 cases of non–small cell lung cancer (NSCLC) to further refine the prognostic accuracy of clinical and pathologic tumor stage.[3] In recent years, however, several prognostic and predictive biomarkers for NSCLC have been identified. Prognostic biomarkers provide information regarding clinical outcomes regardless of therapy.[4] In contrast, predictive biomarkers can be used to indicate potential responsiveness to a therapy or regimen; they can also serve as

The authors have nothing to disclose.
Division of Cardiovascular and Thoracic Surgery, Department of Surgery, Duke University Medical Center, Box 3043, Hock Plaza-2424 Erwin Road, Suite 403, Durham, NC 27710, USA
* Corresponding author.
E-mail address: david.harpole@duke.edu

targets for molecular therapeutic agents.[5] Rather than being either prognostic or predictive, some biomarkers fulfill both roles. This article discusses several key NSCLCs.

INDIVIDUAL GENETIC ALTERATIONS
p53

Alterations in the *p53* tumor suppressor gene are the most frequently found in human cancer; p53 mutations are found in more than half of all human malignancies. More than 90% of small cell lung cancers and up to 50% of NSCLCs harbor deletions or mutations of the *p53* gene.[6,7] The p53 network is quiet and senescent in the normal state. With cellular injury or stress, however, the p53 network is activated. Downstream effects of p53 activation include induction of apoptosis and DNA repair mechanisms as well as cell cycle regulation. Inactivation of *p53* results in overall increased genomic instability and may be manifested as derangements of cell cycle regulation as well as diminished efficiency of DNA repair.[8]

The role of p53 gene mutations and poor survival outcomes has been established. In a prospective study by Ahrendt and colleagues,[9] *p53* gene mutations were independently predictive of decreased survival in stage I tumors. Although missense mutations were not predictive of patient outcomes, mutations that were truncating, structural, or abolishing DNA contact were associated with poorer survival. The relationship between *p53* mutational status and adverse survival outcomes has been corroborated by several other studies incorporating NSCLC samples from all tumor stages.[10–18]

Immunohistochemical studies of p53 have been less consistent. In the largest studies examining p53 expression levels, some investigators have reported a correlation between abnormal p53 expression and poor prognosis; however, others report no statistically significant relationship.[19–27] Despite the mixed evidence from immunohistochemical studies, however, most studies report an association between overexpression of p53 and poorer outcomes. Carbognani and colleagues[28] examined the role of p53 status in long-term survival after surgery for lung adenocarcinoma. Using immunohistochemical analysis and a panel of several potential prognostic markers, p53 status was the only independent predictor of 10-year survival after resection. In another study, Tsao and colleagues[29] observed that p53 protein overexpression was a predictor of both poor prognosis and shorter overall survival (OS). In addition, patients with tumors containing wild-type *p53* had a survival benefit with adjuvant chemotherapy compared with those with functionally aberrant *p53* status. Finally, a systematic review of 56 studies concluded that abnormal *p53* status was associated with decreased OS in patients with NSCLC across all stages and in both squamous cell and adenocarcinoma histologies.[30]

K-ras

The *ras* gene family members encode for cell membrane-associated G proteins, which mediate signal transduction for cellular proliferation. Up to 30% of NSCLCs harbor *K-ras* mutations. The most common mutation in NSCLC is a G → T transversion in codon 12.[31] Activation of *K-ras* results in continuous transmission of growth signals to the nucleus secondary to constitutive activation. *K-ras* mutations are most commonly associated with tumors of adenocarcinoma histology and in patients with a history of tobacco use.[32,33] Up to 15% of tumors in never smokers may harbor *K-ras* mutations; tumor mutations in these patients are often distinct from the G → T and G → C transversions seen in those from smokers.[34] *K-ras* mutations are essentially mutually exclusive with EGFR mutations.

For patients with NSCLC, the prognostic significance of *K-ras* mutations is controversial. Some studies have reported worse prognosis, including decreased survival, in patients whose tumors had *K-ras* mutations.[35] In a small study of patients with advanced NSCLC and *K-ras* mutant tumors, those treated with erlotinib (Tarceva) in addition to chemotherapy had worse outcomes than those with wild-type *K-ras*.[36] Others have reported that tumors with *K-ras* mutations lack sensitivity to either gefitinib (Iressa) or erlotinib.[37] Other studies, however, including a meta-analysis of 881 cases, have reported no significant association between *K-ras* mutation status and clinical outcomes.[7,38,39]

Excision Repair Cross-Complementing 1

The excision repair cross-complementing group 1 (ERCC1) gene product is part of the nucleotide excision repair pathway that recognizes and removes cisplatin-induced DNA adducts.[40,41] Nucleotide excision repair is important in DNA repair and is associated with resistance to chemotherapy with platinum-based agents. Clinically, NSCLC tumors with low ERCC1 expression may demonstrate resistance to cisplatin chemotherapy. In 2002, Lord and colleagues[42] reported that patients with advanced NSCLC whose tumors had low ERCC1 expression had significantly longer OS than those with high ERCC1 expression tumors.

Other studies have confirmed the predictive value of ERCC1 expression. ERCC1 expression was present in 44% of tumors obtained from patients enrolled in the International Adjuvant Lung Cancer Trial.[43] For patients in the trial who were randomized to adjuvant cisplatin-based chemotherapy, those with ERCC1-negative tumors had significantly prolonged survival relative to those who were observed (hazard ratio [HR] 0.65; 95% CI, 0.50–0.86; $P = .002$). There was no survival difference between the observation and chemotherapy for patients with ERCC1-positive tumors.

Furthermore, among those who did not receive adjuvant chemotherapy, patients with ERCC1-positive tumors had improved survival versus those with ERCC1-negative tumors (HR 0.66; 95% CI, 0.49–0.90; $P = 0.009$). Taken together, these results suggest that adjuvant cisplatin-based chemotherapy may benefit patients with ERCC1-negative tumors. Currently, several clinical trials are enrolling patients to further examine the benefit of customized chemotherapy based on ERCC1 status in early-stage (NCT00775385), resected (NCT00792701), and advanced NSCLC (NCT00499109 and NCT00736814).

Cell Cycle Regulatory Genes

Rb and p16
The retinoblastoma susceptibility gene *(Rb),* a tumor suppressor gene with a key role in human carcinogenesis, is inactivated in nearly 90% of small cell lung tumors and 20% to 30% of NSCLCs.[7] Although most studies have reported no significant relationship between *Rb* and lung cancer survival,[20,44–46] there seems to be an additive effect of concurrent abnormalities in the *Rb* and *p53* pathways and it seems that these additive effects are predictive of patient prognosis in NSCLC. In a study by Burke and colleagues,[47] certain combinations of abnormalities were negative predictors of survival: concurrent pRb-negative status and cyclin D1 overexpression; concurrent pRb-negative status, cyclin D1 overexpression, and *p53* mutation; and concurrent cyclin D1 overexpression and *p53* mutation.

The *p16^{INK4A}* gene is a tumor suppressor gene that encodes a cyclin-dependent kinase (CDK) inhibitor. *p16* plays a prominent role in NSCLC; it is inactivated in 40% to 70% of NSCLCs. Under normal circumstances, p16 binds to the cyclin D/CDK4/6 complexes to inhibit phosphorylation of the Rb protein and therefore inhibits cell cycle progression at the G1 → S phase. In a recent study of tumors from patients with stage IIIA NSCLC, the presence of both p16 and p21 proteins correlated with improved long-term survival.[48]

Absent or dysfunctional *p16* expression can result in unchecked progression through the cell cycle. There are several mechanisms of *p16* inactivation, including epigenetic silencing by hypermethylation of the gene promoter CpG island in addition to point mutations or deletions. Alteration and inactivation of *p16* have been associated with metastases, poor prognosis, and decreased OS in patients with NSCLC.[49–52]

The cyclins, p21$^{WAF1/CIP1}$ and p27

Cyclin D1, cyclin E, cyclin B1, *p21$^{WAF1/CIP1}$*, and *p27* are other cell cycle regulatory genes of interest in NSCLC. Up to 47% of NSCLC tumors demonstrate overexpression of cyclin D1; however, the prognostic effects of this overexpression are somewhat controversial. In some studies, favorable outcomes have been associated with overexpression of *cyclin D1*.[53,54] Other studies have reported lymph node metastasis, advanced pathologic stage, and shorter OS in association with this condition.[46,55,56]

Similar results have been reported for *cyclin E* and *cyclin B1*. High levels of *cyclin E* expression, present in up to 53% of NSCLCs, have been correlated with tumor invasion, unfavorable prognosis, and decreased patient survival.[57,58] Overexpression of *cyclin B1* has been linked to shorter survival and seems to occur more commonly in tumors of squamous histology.[59]

p21$^{WAF1/CIP1}$ influences cell cycle progression at multiple sites, binding to several different cyclin/CDK complexes. Some investigators have reported a relationship between p21 expression and improved OS and relapse-free survival, whereas others have found none.[60–63] *p27^{Kip1}* interacts with both cyclin D1 and cyclin E to regulate the cell cycle. Several studies have used immunohistochemical techniques to determine p27 expression. Both overexpression and decreased levels of p27 have been correlated with poor prognosis in NSCLC.[56,64–66]

Gene Arrays

The development and use of gene expression microarrays have facilitated the identification of specific gene signatures that correlate with specific clinical characteristics, such as smoking status and tumor histology.[67–72] Some investigators have used gene expression profiles to predict nodal metastases as well as response to treatment. In a study of 37 NSCLCs, Kikuchi and colleagues[73] used hierarchical clustering methods to establish a predictive scoring system based on the expression profiles of selected genes. With this system, 40 genes were identified whose expression profiles could be used to separate node-positive from node-negative adenocarcinomas.

Many studies have used gene expression arrays to predict overall prognosis and OS. One study used cDNA arrays to examine 39 NSCLC tumors. With unsupervised hierarchical clustering of a subset of 2899 genes, 2 groups were identified that differed significantly in disease-free survival.[74] Similarly, Beer and colleagues[75] examined 86 lung adenocarcinomas using oligonucleotide arrays (HuGeneFL). Using hierarchical clustering and other supervised analytical approaches, 3 clusters of tumors were identified. Significant relationships between clusters and tumor stage and differentiation were observed. Based on this information, a 50-gene risk index based on the top-50 survival-related genes was devised. Using this approach, the investigators were able to predict survival based on the risk index.

Further refinement of gene expression profiling has led to the development of predictive models using few genes. Applying an integrated approach to published gene expression data sets, Bianchi and colleagues[76] described a 10-gene predictive model for OS in stage I lung adenocarcinoma. This model exhibited a prognostic accuracy of 75% validated in 2 independent cohorts.

Similarly, Chen and colleagues[77] used gene expression arrays to develop a 5-gene model for prediction of relapse-free survival and OS in lung cancer. The model was subsequently validated in an independent cohort of 60 additional patients. Compared with those with a low-risk gene signature, patients with a high-risk gene signature had a significantly shorter median survival. When patients were stratified by stage, the model was predictive of survival; however, there was no correlation between gene signature and OS for patients with stage II disease. Further validation studies were performed on 86 tumors previously analyzed by another group.[75] Patients whose tumors exhibited the high-risk gene signature had a significantly higher risk for death from any cause; results for survival trended toward significance.

Finally, Lau and colleagues[78] described a 3-gene signature for predicting prognosis. This model was validated in 2 independent data sets from outside institutions. None of the models (described previously) has genes in common.

TYROSINE KINASES AND TARGETED THERAPIES

Several targeted molecular therapies have been developed for the treatment of NSCLC. Specific targets include the epidermal growth factor receptor (EGFR), vascular endothelial growth factor (VEGF), and anaplastic lymphoma kinase (ALK). Although some agents are approved for use by the US Food and Drug Administration, others are currently under investigation in clinical trials.

Epidermal Growth Factor Receptor

The EGFR family consists of a group of tyrosine kinases whose activation results in a cascade of downstream signals. These signals ultimately lead to enhanced cellular proliferation and angiogenesis and tumor cell mobility as well as diminshed apoptosis.[79] Although rare in small cell lung cancer, EGFR overexpression is common in NSCLC, affecting up to 80% of tumors.[80]

Gefitinib is a selective inhibitor of the EGFR tyrosine kinase with demonstrated clinical benefit in specific populations of patients with NSCLC. In the Iressa Survival Evaluation in Lung Cancer study, treatment with gefitinib as a second-line or third-line treatment did not improve survival in the overall population of patients with advanced NSCLC.[81] There was demonstrated benefit, however, in preplanned subgroup analyses of patients of Asian origin and never-smokers.

EGFR mutation status can also be used to predict response to therapy with EGFR inhibitors. In a recent study of patients with advanced nonsquamous NSCLC, wild-type EGFR was a poor prognostic factor in patients receiving gefitinib therapy.[82] Similarly, in the Iressa Pan-Asia Study, treatment with gefitinib was associated with improved progression-free survival (PFS) (HR 0.74; 95% CI, 0.65–0.85; $P<.001$).[83] Among patients whose tumors harbored EGFR gene mutations, treatment with gefitinib was associated with improved PFS compared with carboplatin-paclitaxel (HR 0.48; 95% CI, −0.36–0.64; $P<.001$). For patients without EGFR mutations, however, PFS was significantly longer in patients treated with carboplatin-paclitaxel (HR for progression or death with gefitinib 2.85; 95% CI, 2.05–3.98; $P<.001$).

Erlotinib, another EGFR inhibitor, is currently used as second-line therapy for locally advanced or metastatic NSCLC. Compared with placebo, patients receiving erlotinib have improved tumor response as well as longer PFS and OS.[84] A recent pooled analysis of more than 60 studies and 1800 patients was conducted to evaluate clinical outcomes in patients with EGFR mutations treated EGFR tyrosine kinase inhibitors (TKIs) versus conventional chemotherapy.[85] Patients treated with gefitinib and erlotinib had longer PFS compared with those treated with chemotherapy (P<.001).

Cetuximab (Erbitux) is a monoclonal antibody targeted against EGFR. These molecules can inhibit ligand binding and receptor activation, thereby inducing apoptosis of tumor cells.[86] Several studies have demonstrated a survival benefit with the addition of cetuximab to standard chemotherapy regimens for patients with advanced NSCLC.

As with other TKIs, however, the efficacy of cetuximab has not been studied in early-stage NSCLC. In a small, randomized phase II study, patients with advanced NSCLC treated with cetuximab plus cisplatin/vinorelbine had improved median survival compared with those in the chemotherapy-alone group.[87] These findings were validated in a larger, phase III randomized trial, in which patients given cisplatin/vinorelbine plus cetuximab survived longer than those in the control group (HR 0.871; 95% CI, 0.762–0.996).[88] Another phase III study of cetuximab plus taxane/carboplatin chemotherapy, however, showed a favorable response rate in patients with advanced NSCLC but failed to demonstrate longer PFS.[89]

Most studies of EGFR TKIs have focused on patients with advanced or recurrent lung cancer; few studies have investigated the use of these agents in the treatment of early-stage or resectable disease. Clinical trials are currently under way, however, to elucidate the role of these agents in conjunction with surgery for stage I-IIIA NSCLC (NCT00104728, NCT00049543, and NCT00324805).

Vascular Endothelial Growth Factor

Bevacizumab (Avastin) is a monoclonal antibody that targets VEGF-A. Its use has been shown to benefit patients with a variety of malignancies, including cancers of the colon, kidney, and brain.[90–92] The presence of VEGF in NSCLC tumors is associated with poor prognosis and OS.[93] The benefit of bevacizumab in NSCLC was demonstrated in a recent phase III study of 878 patients with advanced nonsquamous NSCLC. Patients were randomized to chemotherapy with carboplatin/paclitaxel alone versus chemotherapy with bevacizumab.[94] Those who received bevacizumab in addition to chemotherapy had significantly improved response rates, PFS, and OS. Similarly, in the Avastin in Lung cancer trial, patients were randomized to receive bevacizumab or placebo in addition to chemotherapy with cisplatin/gemcitabine.[95] Although OS was not different between the 2 groups, PFS was significantly prolonged with the addition of bevacizumab compared with placebo. The risk of progression or death at any time was reduced by 25% in the bevacizumab group (HR 0.75; 95% CI, 0.64–0.87; P = .0003).

A potential role of bevacizumab in the treatment of early-stage (IB-IIIA) lung cancer is under investigation in the Eastern Cooperative Oncology Group E1505 adjuvant therapy trial (NCT00324805). In this phase III study, patients with resected NSCLC are randomized to one of 4 adjuvant chemotherapy regimens, with or without bevacizumab. In addition to OS and disease-free survival, tissue and blood specimens are being collected to identify factors predictive of clinical outcomes.

Anaplastic Lymphoma Kinase

In 2007, Soda and colleagues[96] identified the fusion gene of echinoderm microtubule-associated protein-like 4 (EML4) and ALK in a subset of NSCLCs. These EML4-ALK fusion products are present in 3% to 13% of NSCLCs. Perhaps more interesting is that they are mutually exclusive to tumors with EGFR mutations.[97] Other clinical features associated with EML4-ALK fusions include younger age, male gender, light-smoking or never-smoking status, adenocarcinoma (specifically acinar) histology, and negative *K-ras* mutational status.[98–101]

Crizotinib is an oral selective inhibitor of the ALK and MET tyrosine kinases. In recent studies, the use of crizotinib for patients with advanced ALK-positive NSCLC was associated with a clinical benefit, defined as tumor response plus stable disease.[89,102] Currently, these agents are limited to use in patients with advanced NSCLC. Studies are being conducted, however, to evaluate the usefulness of these targeted molecular therapies. One study is investigating the use of crizotinib as standard therapy in patients with documented EML4-ALK mutations (NCT01154140); another is examining usefulness of crizotinib in combination with traditional chemotherapeutic agents in the neoadjuvant setting (NCT00924209).

PROTEOMICS

Proteomic approaches are used to characterize tumors based on protein expressions. Profiling is done using either 2-D polyacrylamide gel electrophoresis or liquid chromatography coupled to tandem mass spectrometry (LC-MS/MS). In contrast to genomic approaches, one advantage of proteomic analysis is the ability to study post-translational modification of proteins, including proteolytic processing, glycosylation, and phosphorylation.

The use of proteomics to profile tumors and predict outcomes has been described in both early-stage and advanced-stage lung tumors.[103] In a recent study of patients with resected stage I adenocarcinoma, LC-MS was used to detect the presence of myosin IIA and vimentin, with expression and distribution confirmed by immunohistochemistry.[104] Patients with tumors lacking expression of either protein had significantly better survival outcomes than those whose tumors expressed either vimentin or both proteins, regardless of adjuvant chemotherapy. Investigators of another study used proteomic evaluation to classify lung cancer versus benign lung disease with 93.1% diagnostic accuracy using patterns of differentially expressed peaks.[105] In addition, they identified a 4628-Da protein that was independently and significantly associated with prognosis in patients with advanced NSCLC.

Recently, proteomic profiling has been used to predict outcomes for patients with NSCLC. In one study of patients with advanced NSCLC previously treated with EGFR TKIs, an 8-peak predictive algorithm was developed based on analysis of patient serum.[106] Although not predictive of outcomes with other regimens, this 8-peak signature specifically and successfully predicted patient response to TKIs. In another study of 105 tumor samples, improved OS was seen in tumors demonstrating overexpression of the glucocorticoid receptor.[107] Although these studies demonstrate the usefulness of proteomics for molecular prognostication for patients with lung cancer, there are currently no proteomic-based targeted therapies under investigation, especially for early-stage disease.

MICRORNAs

MicroRNAs (miRNAs) were initially discovered in *Caenorhabditis elegans*[108] They are noncoding fragments of RNA, measuring 18 to 25 nucleotides long, that play a role in regulating cellular processes, such as cell development, metabolism, proliferation, and even cell death.[109] MiRNAs can increase the stability of mRNA or even regulate mRNA translation, thereby altering the amount of final product.[110] Currently, the role of miRNAs in human carcinogenesis has yet to be completely defined. Several studies have demonstrated, however, abnormal expression of miRNA in human malignancies, including lung cancer.[111,112]

Several specific miRNAs and miRNA families have been studied in lung cancer. The *lethal-7* (*let-7*) miRNA family is abundantly expressed in normal human lung tissue, and at least one member of the *let-7* family has been shown to negatively regulate *RAS* expression in human cells.[111] Reduced *let-7* miRNA expression has been associated with poor prognosis and shorter long-term survival, independent of disease stage.[113,114] Similarly, members of the miR-34 family are part of the p53 network, with expression directly induced by p53. Diminished miR-34a expression has been demonstrated in NSCLC tumor tissue, and patients with low miR-34a are at significantly higher risk of recurrence.[115] Other miRNAs associated with lung cancer include the miR-29 family, miR-21, miR-221, miE-222, miR-210, and miR-451.[112]

Unique miRNA expression profiles have been described for NSCLC. Several studies have correlated specific miRNA profiles with patient survival. Comparing lung tumors to noncancerous lung, Yanaihara and colleagues[114] identified 43 miRNAs that were differentially expressed in tumor tissue. Six of these miRNAs were expressed differently between tumors of adenocarcinoma versus squamous histology. In addition, for patients with adenocarcinoma, up-regulation and down-regulation of specific miRNAs was associated with a significantly worse prognosis, independent of other clinicopathologic variables. In another study, Yu and colleagues[116] identified a 5-miRNA signature from a cohort of 56 NSCLC tumors with both adenocarcinoma and squamous cell histologies. Based on the expression levels of 5 miRNAs, a risk-score formula was devised. Significantly shorter median relapse-free survival and OS times were noted for patients whose tumors had high-risk miRNA signatures, independent of tumor histology. The investigators validated these findings using an independent set of samples. In a recent study of tumors from patients enrolled in the International Adjuvant Lung Cancer Trial, however, expression levels of 5 biologically relevant miRNAs were examined.[117] Of these, only decreased expression of miR-21 was found to be associated with decreased survival.

PERSONALIZED LUNG CANCER TREATMENT—CURRENT TRIALS

Several randomized trials are currently under way to investigate the possibility of "customized" adjuvant chemotherapy regimens for patients with resected NSCLC. These trials incorporate the use of standard chemotherapy regimens with testing for specific biomarkers. Patients in the experimental arms receive targeted biologic therapies, either in addition to or in lieu of standard chemotherapy regimens. Positive results from these studies would further emphasize the potential benefit and usefulness of individualized therapy for patients with NSCLC.

The TAilored Post-Surgical Therapy in Early Stage NSCLC (NCT00775385) trial is a randomized study of patients with nonsquamous, resected stages II and IIIA (non-N2) NSCLC. After resection, patients' tumors will be tested for both ERCC1 and EGFR mutations. Those in the experimental arm with EGFR mutations will receive erlotinib as customized chemotherapy. Treatment of those with wild-type EGFR will depend on ERCC1 levels: (1) patients whose tumors exhibit high ERCC1 levels will receive no adjuvant therapy and (2) those with low ERCC1 levels assigned to receive 4 cycles of adjuvant cisplatin and pemetrexed.

Similarly, the Southwest Oncology Group S0720 Trial (NCT00792701) is studying the role of ERCC1 and the ribonucleotide reductase M1 (RRM1), which provides deoxyribonucleotides for DNA repair as well as de novo DNA synthesis.[118] RRM1 is inhibited by gemcitabine. Patients with surgically resected stage IA or IB NSCLC are tested for ERCC1 and RRM1 levels. Given the expected favorable prognosis, those with high levels of ERCC1 and RRM1 are assigned to active surveillance.

With expected poorer prognosis, patients with low expression levels of either ERCC1 or RRM1 are assigned to adjuvant chemotherapy with gemcitabine and cisplatin.

SUMMARY

The successful treatment of lung cancer remains elusive for many patients. The development and use of molecular techniques, however, has significantly increased clinicians' armamentarium for both treatment and prognostication of lung cancer. Although molecular-based treatments are now standard for advanced NSCLC, the use of targeted therapies, such as TKIs and monoclonal antibodies, as well as individual genomic and proteomic signatures in the treatment of early-stage NSCLC is emerging. Several randomized clinical trials are currently in progress and should provide interesting results in the near future.

REFERENCES

1. American Cancer Society. Cancer facts & figures. Atlanta: American Cancer Society; 2011. 2011.
2. Parkin DM. Global cancer statistics in the year 2000. Lancet Oncol 2001;2(9): 533–43.
3. Goldstraw P, Crowley J, Chansky K, et al. The IASLC Lung Cancer Staging Project: proposals for the revision of the TNM stage groupings in the forthcoming (seventh) edition of the TNM classification of malignant tumours. J Thorac Oncol 2007;2(8):706–14.
4. Perez-Soler R. Individualized therapy in non-small-cell lung cancer: future versus current clinical practice. Oncogene 2009;28(Suppl 1):S38–45.
5. Oldenhuis CN, Oosting SF, Gietema JA, et al. Prognostic versus predictive value of biomarkers in oncology. Eur J Cancer 2008;44(7):946–53.
6. Ahrendt SA, Chow JT, Yang SC, et al. Alcohol consumption and cigarette smoking increase the frequency of p53 mutations in non-small cell lung cancer. Cancer Res 2000;60(12):3155–9.
7. Fischer JR, Lahm H. Validation of molecular and immunological factors with predictive importance in lung cancer. Lung Cancer 2004;45(Suppl 2):S151–61.
8. Vogelstein B, Lane D, Levine AJ. Surfing the p53 network. Nature 2000; 408(6810):307–10.
9. Ahrendt SA, Hu Y, Buta M, et al. p53 mutations and survival in stage I non-small-cell lung cancer: results of a prospective study. J Natl Cancer Inst 2003;95(13): 961–70.
10. Fukuyama Y, Mitsudomi T, Sugio K, et al. K-ras and p53 mutations are an independent unfavourable prognostic indicator in patients with non-small-cell lung cancer. Br J Cancer 1997;75(8):1125–30.
11. Hashimoto T, Tokuchi Y, Hayashi M, et al. p53 null mutations undetected by immunohistochemical staining predict a poor outcome with early-stage non-small cell lung carcinomas. Cancer Res 1999;59(21):5572–7.
12. Horio Y, Takahashi T, Kuroishi T, et al. Prognostic significance of p53 mutations and 3p deletions in primary resected non-small cell lung cancer. Cancer Res 1993;53(1):1–4.
13. Huang CL, Taki T, Adachi M, et al. Mutations of p53 and K-ras genes as prognostic factors for non-small cell lung cancer. Int J Oncol 1998;12(3):553–63.
14. Laudanski J, Niklinska W, Burzykowski T, et al. Prognostic significance of p53 and bcl-2 abnormalities in operable nonsmall cell lung cancer. Eur Respir J 2001;17(4):660–6.

15. Mitsudomi T, Oyama T, Kusano T, et al. Mutations of the p53 gene as a predictor of poor prognosis in patients with non-small-cell lung cancer. J Natl Cancer Inst 1993;85(24):2018–23.

16. Skaug V, Ryberg D, Kure EH, et al. p53 mutations in defined structural and functional domains are related to poor clinical outcome in non-small cell lung cancer patients. Clin Cancer Res 2000;6(3):1031–7.

17. Tomizawa Y, Kohno T, Fujita T, et al. Correlation between the status of the p53 gene and survival in patients with stage I non-small cell lung carcinoma. Oncogene 1999;18(4):1007–14.

18. Vega FJ, Iniesta P, Caldes T, et al. p53 exon 5 mutations as a prognostic indicator of shortened survival in non-small-cell lung cancer. Br J Cancer 1997;76(1):44–51.

19. Dalquen P, Sauter G, Torhorst J, et al. Nuclear p53 overexpression is an independent prognostic parameter in node-negative non-small cell lung carcinoma. J Pathol 1996;178(1):53–8.

20. D'Amico TA, Massey M, Herndon JE 2nd, et al. A biologic risk model for stage I lung cancer: immunohistochemical analysis of 408 patients with the use of ten molecular markers. J Thorac Cardiovasc Surg 1999;117(4):736–43.

21. Harpole DH Jr, Herndon JE 2nd, Wolfe WG, et al. A prognostic model of recurrence and death in stage I non-small cell lung cancer utilizing presentation, histopathology, and oncoprotein expression. Cancer Res 1995;55(1): 51–6.

22. Kwiatkowski DJ, Harpole DH Jr, Godleski J, et al. Molecular pathologic substaging in 244 stage I non-small-cell lung cancer patients: clinical implications. J Clin Oncol 1998;16(7):2468–77.

23. Lee YC, Chang YL, Luh SP, et al. Significance of P53 and Rb protein expression in surgically treated non-small cell lung cancers. Ann Thorac Surg 1999;68(2): 343–7 [discussion: 348].

24. Moldvay J, Scheid P, Wild P, et al. Predictive survival markers in patients with surgically resected non-small cell lung carcinoma. Clin Cancer Res 2000;6(3): 1125–34.

25. Nishio M, Koshikawa T, Kuroishi T, et al. Prognostic significance of abnormal p53 accumulation in primary, resected non-small-cell lung cancers. J Clin Oncol 1996;14(2):497–502.

26. Pappot H, Francis D, Brunner N, et al. p53 protein in non-small cell lung cancer as quantitated by enzyme-linked immunosorbent assay: relation to prognosis. Clin Cancer Res 1996;2(1):155–60.

27. Pastorino U, Andreola S, Tagliabue E, et al. Immunocytochemical markers in stage I lung cancer: relevance to prognosis. J Clin Oncol 1997;15(8): 2858–65.

28. Carbognani P, Tincani G, Crafa P, et al. Biological markers in non-small cell lung cancer. Retrospective study of 10 year follow-up after surgery. J Cardiovasc Surg (Torino) 2002;43(4):545–8.

29. Tsao MS, Aviel-Ronen S, Ding K, et al. Prognostic and predictive importance of p53 and RAS for adjuvant chemotherapy in non small-cell lung cancer. J Clin Oncol 2007;25(33):5240–7.

30. Steels E, Paesmans M, Berghmans T, et al. Role of p53 as a prognostic factor for survival in lung cancer: a systematic review of the literature with a meta-analysis. Eur Respir J 2001;18(4):705–19.

31. Breuer RH, Postmus PE, Smit EF. Molecular pathology of non-small-cell lung cancer. Respiration 2005;72(3):313–30.

32. Ahrendt SA, Decker PA, Alawi EA, et al. Cigarette smoking is strongly associated with mutation of the K-ras gene in patients with primary adenocarcinoma of the lung. Cancer 2001;92(6):1525–30.
33. Webb JD, Simon MC. Novel insights into the molecular origins and treatment of lung cancer. Cell Cycle 2010;9(20):4098–105.
34. Riely GJ, Kris MG, Rosenbaum D, et al. Frequency and distinctive spectrum of KRAS mutations in never smokers with lung adenocarcinoma. Clin Cancer Res 2008;14(18):5731–4.
35. Nelson HH, Christiani DC, Mark EJ, et al. Implications and prognostic value of K-ras mutation for early-stage lung cancer in women. J Natl Cancer Inst 1999; 91(23):2032–8.
36. Eberhard DA, Johnson BE, Amler LC, et al. Mutations in the epidermal growth factor receptor and in KRAS are predictive and prognostic indicators in patients with non-small-cell lung cancer treated with chemotherapy alone and in combination with erlotinib. J Clin Oncol 2005;23(25):5900–9.
37. Pao W, Wang TY, Riely GJ, et al. KRAS mutations and primary resistance of lung adenocarcinomas to gefitinib or erlotinib. PLoS Med 2005;2(1):e17.
38. Huncharek M, Muscat J, Geschwind JF. K-ras oncogene mutation as a prognostic marker in non-small cell lung cancer: a combined analysis of 881 cases. Carcinogenesis 1999;20(8):1507–10.
39. Vielh P, Spano JP, Grenier J, et al. Molecular prognostic factors in resectable non-small cell lung cancer. Crit Rev Oncol Hematol 2005;53(3):193–7.
40. Simon GR, Sharma S, Cantor A, et al. ERCC1 expression is a predictor of survival in resected patients with non-small cell lung cancer. Chest 2005; 127(3):978–83.
41. Ikeda N, Nagase S, Ohira T. Individualized adjuvant chemotherapy for surgically resected lung cancer and the roles of biomarkers. Ann Thorac Cardiovasc Surg 2009;15(3):144–9.
42. Lord RV, Brabender J, Gandara D, et al. Low ERCC1 expression correlates with prolonged survival after cisplatin plus gemcitabine chemotherapy in non-small cell lung cancer. Clin Cancer Res 2002;8(7):2286–91.
43. Olaussen KA, Dunant A, Fouret P, et al. DNA repair by ERCC1 in non-small-cell lung cancer and cisplatin-based adjuvant chemotherapy. N Engl J Med 2006; 355(10):983–91.
44. Akin H, Yilmazbayhan D, Kilicaslan Z, et al. Clinical significance of P16INK4A and retinoblastoma proteins in non-small-cell lung carcinoma. Lung Cancer 2002;38(3):253–60.
45. Haga Y, Hiroshima K, Iyoda A, et al. Ki-67 expression and prognosis for smokers with resected stage I non-small cell lung cancer. Ann Thorac Surg 2003;75(6): 1727–32 [discussion: 1732–3].
46. Jin M, Inoue S, Umemura T, et al. Cyclin D1, p16 and retinoblastoma gene product expression as a predictor for prognosis in non-small cell lung cancer at stages I and II. Lung Cancer 2001;34(2):207–18.
47. Burke L, Flieder DB, Guinee DG, et al. Prognostic implications of molecular and immunohistochemical profiles of the Rb and p53 cell cycle regulatory pathways in primary non-small cell lung carcinoma. Clin Cancer Res 2005;11(1):232–41.
48. Mohamed S, Yasufuku K, Hiroshima K, et al. Prognostic implications of cell cycle-related proteins in primary resectable pathologic N2 nonsmall cell lung cancer. Cancer 2007;109(12):2506–14.
49. Groeger AM, Caputi M, Esposito V, et al. Independent prognostic role of p16 expression in lung cancer. J Thorac Cardiovasc Surg 1999;118(3):529–35.

50. Huang CI, Taki T, Higashiyama M, et al. p16 protein expression is associated with a poor prognosis in squamous cell carcinoma of the lung. Br J Cancer 2000;82(2):374–80.

51. Kawabuchi B, Moriyama S, Hironaka M, et al. p16 inactivation in small-sized lung adenocarcinoma: its association with poor prognosis. Int J Cancer 1999; 84(1):49–53.

52. Kratzke RA, Greatens TM, Rubins JB, et al. Rb and p16INK4a expression in resected non-small cell lung tumors. Cancer Res 1996;56(15):3415–20.

53. Gugger M, Kappeler A, Vonlanthen S, et al. Alterations of cell cycle regulators are less frequent in advanced non-small cell lung cancer than in resectable tumours. Lung Cancer 2001;33(2–3):229–39.

54. Nishio M, Koshikawa T, Yatabe Y, et al. Prognostic significance of cyclin D1 and retinoblastoma expression in combination with p53 abnormalities in primary, resected non-small cell lung cancers. Clin Cancer Res 1997;3(7):1051–8.

55. Keum JS, Kong G, Yang SC, et al. Cyclin D1 overexpression is an indicator of poor prognosis in resectable non-small cell lung cancer. Br J Cancer 1999; 81(1):127–32.

56. Sterlacci W, Fiegl M, Hilbe W, et al. Deregulation of p27 and cyclin D1/D3 control over mitosis is associated with unfavorable prognosis in non-small cell lung cancer, as determined in 405 operated patients. J Thorac Oncol 2010;5(9):1325–36.

57. Fukuse T, Hirata T, Naiki H, et al. Prognostic significance of cyclin E overexpression in resected non-small cell lung cancer. Cancer Res 2000;60(2):242–4.

58. Mishina T, Dosaka-Akita H, Hommura F, et al. Cyclin E expression, a potential prognostic marker for non-small cell lung cancers. Clin Cancer Res 2000;6(1):11–6.

59. Soria JC, Rodriguez M, Liu DD, et al. Aberrant promoter methylation of multiple genes in bronchial brush samples from former cigarette smokers. Cancer Res 2002;62(2):351–5.

60. Esposito V, Baldi A, De Luca A, et al. Prognostic role of the cyclin-dependent kinase inhibitor p27 in non-small cell lung cancer. Cancer Res 1997;57(16): 3381–5.

61. Komiya T, Hosono Y, Hirashima T, et al. p21 expression as a predictor for favorable prognosis in squamous cell carcinoma of the lung. Clin Cancer Res 1997; 3(10):1831–5.

62. Shoji T, Tanaka F, Takata T, et al. Clinical significance of p21 expression in non-small-celllung cancer. J Clin Oncol 2002;20(18):3865–71.

63. Wu DW, Liu WS, Wang J, et al. Reduced p21(WAF1/CIP1) via alteration of p53-DDX3 pathway is associated with poor relapse-free survival in early-stage human papillomavirus-associated lung cancer. Clin Cancer Res 2011;17(7): 1895–905.

64. Hayashi H, Ogawa N, Ishiwa N, et al. High cyclin E and low p27/Kip1 expressions are potentially poor prognostic factors in lung adenocarcinoma patients. Lung Cancer 2001;34(1):59–65.

65. Hommura F, Dosaka-Akita H, Mishina T, et al. Prognostic significance of p27KIP1 protein and ki-67 growth fraction in non-small cell lung cancers. Clin Cancer Res 2000;6(10):4073–81.

66. Tsukamoto S, Sugio K, Sakada T, et al. Reduced expression of cell-cycle regulator p27(Kip1) correlates with a shortened survival in non-small cell lung cancer. Lung Cancer 2001;34(1):83–90.

67. Bhattacharjee A, Richards WG, Staunton J, et al. Classification of human lung carcinomas by mRNA expression profiling reveals distinct adenocarcinoma subclasses. Proc Natl Acad Sci U S A 2001;98(24):13790–5.

68. Borczuk AC, Toonkel RL, Powell CA. Genomics of lung cancer. Proc Am Thorac Soc 2009;6(2):152–8.
69. Campioni M, Ambrogi V, Pompeo E, et al. Identification of genes down-regulated during lung cancer progression: a cDNA array study. J Exp Clin Cancer Res 2008;27:38.
70. Hayes DN, Monti S, Parmigiani G, et al. Gene expression profiling reveals repro-ducible human lung adenocarcinoma subtypes in multiple independent patient cohorts. J Clin Oncol 2006;24(31):5079–90.
71. Lerman MI, Minna JD. The 630-kb lung cancer homozygous deletion region on human chromosome 3p21.3: identification and evaluation of the resident candi-date tumor suppressor genes. The International Lung Cancer Chromosome 3p21.3 Tumor Suppressor Gene Consortium. Cancer Res 2000;60(21):6116–33.
72. Miura K, Bowman ED, Simon R, et al. Laser capture microdissection and micro-array expression analysis of lung adenocarcinoma reveals tobacco smoking-and prognosis-related molecular profiles. Cancer Res 2002;62(11):3244–50.
73. Kikuchi T, Daigo Y, Katagiri T, et al. Expression profiles of non-small cell lung cancers on cDNA microarrays: identification of genes for prediction of lymph-node metastasis and sensitivity to anti-cancer drugs. Oncogene 2003;22(14):2192–205.
74. Wigle DA, Jurisica I, Radulovich N, et al. Molecular profiling of non-small cell lung cancer and correlation with disease-free survival. Cancer Res 2002;62(11):3005–8.
75. Beer DG, Kardia SL, Huang CC, et al. Gene-expression profiles predict survival of patients with lung adenocarcinoma. Nat Med 2002;8(8):816–24.
76. Bianchi F, Nuciforo P, Vecchi M, et al. Survival prediction of stage I lung adeno-carcinomas by expression of 10 genes. J Clin Invest 2007;117(11):3436–44.
77. Chen HY, Yu SL, Chen CH, et al. A five-gene signature and clinical outcome in non-small-cell lung cancer. N Engl J Med 2007;356(1):11–20.
78. Lau SK, Boutros PC, Pintilie M, et al. Three-gene prognostic classifier for early-stage non small-cell lung cancer. J Clin Oncol 2007;25(35):5562–9.
79. Scagliotti GV, Selvaggi G, Novello S, et al. The biology of epidermal growth factor receptor in lung cancer. Clin Cancer Res 2004;10(12 Pt 2):4227s–32s.
80. Johnson BE, Janne PA. Epidermal growth factor receptor mutations in patients with non-small cell lung cancer. Cancer Res 2005;65(17):7525–9.
81. Thatcher N, Chang A, Parikh P, et al. Gefitinib plus best supportive care in previ-ously treated patients with refractory advanced non-small-cell lung cancer: results from a randomised, placebo-controlled, multicentre study (Iressa Survival Evaluation in Lung Cancer). Lancet 2005;366(9496):1527–37.
82. Masago K, Fujita S, Togashi Y, et al. Clinical significance of epidermal growth factor receptor mutations and insulin-like growth factor 1 and its binding protein 3 in advanced non-squamous non-small cell lung cancer. Oncol Rep 2011;26(4):795–803.
83. Mok TS, Wu YL, Thongprasert S, et al. Gefitinib or carboplatin-paclitaxel in pulmonary adenocarcinoma. N Engl J Med 2009;361(10):947–57.
84. Johnson JR, Cohen M, Sridhara R, et al. Approval summary for erlotinib for treat-ment of patients with locally advanced or metastatic non-small cell lung cancer after failure of at least one prior chemotherapy regimen. Clin Cancer Res 2005;11(18):6414–21.
85. Paz-Ares L, Soulieres D, Melezinek I, et al. Clinical outcomes in non-small-cell lung cancer patients with EGFR mutations: pooled analysis. J Cell Mol Med 2010;14(1–2):51–69.

86. Baselga J, Arteaga CL. Critical update and emerging trends in epidermal growth factor receptor targeting in cancer. J Clin Oncol 2005;23(11):2445–59.

87. Rosell R, Robinet G, Szczesna A, et al. Randomized phase II study of cetuximab plus cisplatin/vinorelbine compared with cisplatin/vinorelbine alone as first-line therapy in EGFR-expressing advanced non-small-cell lung cancer. Ann Oncol 2008;19(2):362–9.

88. Pirker R, Pereira JR, Szczesna A, et al. Cetuximab plus chemotherapy in patients with advanced non-small-cell lung cancer (FLEX): an open-label randomised phase III trial. Lancet 2009;373(9674):1525–31.

89. Kwak EL, Bang YJ, Camidge DR, et al. Anaplastic lymphoma kinase inhibition in non-small-cell lung cancer. N Engl J Med 2010;363(18):1693–703.

90. Desjardins A, Reardon DA, Coan A, et al. Bevacizumab and daily temozolomide for recurrent glioblastoma. Cancer 2011 Jul 26. [Epub ahead of print]. DOI: 10.1002/cncr.26381.

91. Hutson TE. Targeted therapies for the treatment of metastatic renal cell carcinoma: clinical evidence. Oncologist 2011;16(Suppl 2):14–22.

92. Pal SK, Figlin RA, Reckamp K. Targeted therapies for non-small cell lung cancer: an evolving landscape. Mol Cancer Ther 2010;9(7):1931–44.

93. Singhal S, Vachani A, Antin-Ozerkis D, et al. Prognostic implications of cell cycle, apoptosis, and angiogenesis biomarkers in non-small cell lung cancer: a review. Clin Cancer Res 2005;11(11):3974–86.

94. Sandler A, Gray R, Perry MC, et al. Paclitaxel-carboplatin alone or with bevacizumab for non-small-cell lung cancer. N Engl J Med 2006;355(24):2542–50.

95. Reck M, von Pawel J, Zatloukal P, et al. Overall survival with cisplatin-gemcitabine and bevacizumab or placebo as first-line therapy for nonsquamous non-small-cell lung cancer: results from a randomised phase III trial (AVAiL). Ann Oncol: official journal of the European Society for Medical Oncology/ESMO 2010;21(9): 1804–9.

96. Soda M, Choi YL, Enomoto M, et al. Identification of the transforming EML4-ALK fusion gene in non-small-cell lung cancer. Nature 2007;448(7153):561–6.

97. Sasaki T, Rodig SJ, Chirieac LR, et al. The biology and treatment of EML4-ALK non-small cell lung cancer. Eur J Cancer 2010;46(10):1773–80.

98. Koivunen JP, Mermel C, Zejnullahu K, et al. EML4-ALK fusion gene and efficacy of an ALK kinase inhibitor in lung cancer. Clin Cancer Res 2008;14(13):4275–83.

99. Wong DW, Leung EL, So KK, et al. The EML4-ALK fusion gene is involved in various histologic types of lung cancers from nonsmokers with wild-type EGFR and KRAS. Cancer 2009;115(8):1723–33.

100. Inamura K, Takeuchi K, Togashi Y, et al. EML4-ALK lung cancers are characterized by rare other mutations, a TTF-1 cell lineage, an acinar histology, and young onset. Mod Pathol 2009;22(4):508–15.

101. Martelli MP, Sozzi G, Hernandez L, et al. EML4-ALK rearrangement in non-small cell lung cancer and non-tumor lung tissues. Am J Pathol 2009;174(2):661–70.

102. Ou SH, Bazhenova L, Camidge DR, et al. Rapid and dramatic radiographic and clinical response to an ALK inhibitor (crizotinib, PF02341066) in an ALK translocation-positive patient with non-small cell lung cancer. J Thorac Oncol 2010;5(12):2044–6.

103. Lehtio J, De Petris L. Lung cancer proteomics, clinical and technological considerations. J Proteomics 2010;73(10):1851–63.

104. Maeda J, Hirano T, Ogiwara A, et al. Proteomic analysis of stage I primary lung adenocarcinoma aimed at individualisation of postoperative therapy. Br J Cancer 2008;98(3):596–603.

105. Jacot W, Lhermitte L, Dossat N, et al. Serum proteomic profiling of lung cancer in high-risk groups and determination of clinical outcomes. J Thorac Oncol 2008;3(8):840–50.
106. Taguchi F, Solomon B, Gregorc V, et al. Mass spectrometry to classify non-small-cell lung cancer patients for clinical outcome after treatment with epidermal growth factor receptor tyrosine kinase inhibitors: a multicohort cross-institutional study. J Natl Cancer Inst 2007;99(11):838–46.
107. Surati M, Robinson M, Nandi S, et al. Proteomic characterization of non-small cell lung cancer in a comprehensive translational thoracic oncology database. J Clin Bioinforma 2011;1(8):1–11.
108. Lee RC, Feinbaum RL, Ambros V. The C. elegans heterochronic gene lin-4 encodes small RNAs with antisense complementarity to lin-14. Cell 1993; 75(5):843–54.
109. Calin GA, Croce CM. MicroRNA signatures in human cancers. Nat Rev Cancer 2006;6(11):857–66.
110. Eder M, Scherr M. MicroRNA and lung cancer. N Engl J Med 2005;352(23): 2446–8.
111. Johnson SM, Grosshans H, Shingara J, et al. RAS is regulated by the let-7 microRNA family. Cell 2005;120(5):635–47.
112. Markou A, Liang Y, Lianidou E. Review: prognostic, therapeutic and diagnostic potential of microRNAs in non-small cell lung cancer. Clin Chem Lab Med 2011 Jul 18. [Epub ahead of print].
113. Takamizawa J, Konishi H, Yanagisawa K, et al. Reduced expression of the let-7 microRNAs in human lung cancers in association with shortened postoperative survival. Cancer Res 2004;64(11):3753–6.
114. Yanaihara N, Caplen N, Bowman E, et al. Unique microRNA molecular profiles in lung cancer diagnosis and prognosis. Cancer Cell 2006;9(3):189–98.
115. Gallardo E, Navarro A, Vinolas N, et al. miR-34a as a prognostic marker of relapse in surgically resected non-small-cell lung cancer. Carcinogenesis 2009;30(11):1903–9.
116. Yu SL, Chen HY, Chang GC, et al. MicroRNA signature predicts survival and relapse in lung cancer. Cancer Cell 2008;13(1):48–57.
117. Voortman J, Goto A, Mendiboure J, et al. MicroRNA expression and clinical outcomes in patients treated with adjuvant chemotherapy after complete resection of non-small cell lung carcinoma. Cancer Res 2010;70(21):8288–98.
118. Sangha R, Price J, Butts CA. Adjuvant therapy in non-small cell lung cancer: current and future directions. Oncologist 2010;15(8):862–72.

Index

Note: Page numbers of article titles are in **boldface** type.

A

Adenocarcinoma, gastric. *See also* Gastric cancer.
 D2 nodal dissection for **57–70**
Adjuvant therapy, for gastric cancer, impact of D2 dissection on results of, 75
 strategies in gastric cancer, 100–105
  chemoradiation, 101–102
  chemotherapy, 102–103
  perioperative chemotherapy, 103–105
 targeted, of gastrointestinal stromal tumor of stomach, 25–27
Anaplasma lymphoma kinase, in targeted therapy of lung cancer, 166–167
Angiogenesis inhibitors, clinical trials in advanced gastric cancer, 115–118
  monoclonal antibodies, 116–117
  receptor tyrosine kinase inhibitors, 117–118
Asia, gastric cancer in. *See* Eastern experience.

B

Breast cancer, managing risk of lobular, in hereditary diffuse gastric cancer, 51

C

CDH1 genetic testing, for hereditary diffuse gastric cancer, 45–46
  minimum age for, 46–47
Cell cycle inhibitors, in gastric cancer therapy, 122
Cell cycle regulatory genes, individual genetic alteration as marker in lung cancer, 163–164
Chemoradiation, adjuvant, for gastric cancer, 101–102
 neoadjuvant, for gastric cancer, 105–106
Chemotherapy, clinical trials in advanced gastric cancer, 114–115
 preoperative and postoperative for gastric cancer, **99–112**
  adjuvant strategies, 100–105
  neoadjuvant strategies, 105–106
  ongoing trials, 107–108
  rationale for, 100
  selection of treatment strategy, 106–107
  treatment planning and surgery, 100
Classification, of gastric cancer, role of endoscopy in, 1–3
CLEAN-NET, full-layer resection for gastric cancer with, 135–139
Clinical trials. *See* Trials.

D

D1 nodal dissection, trials in gastric cancer, 84–88
D2 nodal dissection, for gastric cancer, impact on results of adjuvant therapy, 75–76

Surg Oncol Clin N Am 21 (2012) 177–185
doi:10.1016/S1055-3207(11)00090-1
1055-3207/12/$ – see front matter © 2012 Elsevier Inc. All rights reserved.
surgonc.theclinics.com

Moving?

Make sure your subscription moves with you!

To notify us of your new address, find your **Clinics Account Number** (located on your mailing label above your name), and contact customer service at:

Email: journalscustomerservice-usa@elsevier.com

800-654-2452 (subscribers in the U.S. & Canada)
314-447-8871 (subscribers outside of the U.S. & Canada)

Fax number: 314-447-8029

Elsevier Health Sciences Division
Subscription Customer Service
3251 Riverport Lane
Maryland Heights, MO 63043